LAYMAN'S MEDICAL DICTIONARY

Allergy: What It Is and What to Do about It
Your Hay Fever and What to Do about It
The Allergic Child

Frederick Ungar Publishing Co.

New York

ENLARGED EDITION

LAYMAN'S

MEDICAL

DICTIONARY

with plates and tables

HARRY SWARTZ, M.D.

First published as
Intelligent Layman's Medical Dictionary

for E. S. M. and L. G.

The doctor is most effective when those around him—and this group certainly includes his patients—have an immediate understanding of the words and terms that he uses. In the prolonging and saving of human life, the science of communication has been ignored—perhaps for too long. To know precisely what an ailment is, and thus to realize clearly what the requirements of the curative measures are, places the doctor and those around him in the position of working as a team. The objective toward which this team strives is one of the finest ideals of civilized man. In order to function as an efficient working unit, the members of this team—the doctor's secretary, his technician, the nurse, the orderly in the hospital, the volunteer worker, the practical nurse in the home, the patient, the patient's family—must be able to communicate with one another simply and easily. It is indeed a pity that through obscurity of language persons who should be staunch friends in a noble enterprise are instead often confused and bewildered.

Such ease of communication is of great importance also in the dissemination of newer medical knowledge. The accuracy of such knowledge released to the public at large through the medical journalist, the newspaper reporter and editor, television and radio commentators, is often vital to those receiving it.

Generally, in the broad area of human relations, since illness is ubiquitous in both time and place, ease of communication in the language that has grown up about it is of primary importance. The lawyer and his client involved in a compensable illness or injury; the personnel director in judging employability; the employer in understanding employee health needs—all of these and many in other relationships require a clear understanding of the simpler medical language.

The purpose of this *Intelligent Layman's Medical Dictionary* is simply to express in everyday language those medical, anatomical, surgical, and psychiatric terms that are so meaningful in the struggle in which we are all involved, for a richer, fuller, more satisfying life.

In order to maintain the simplicity of this volume and at the same time to make it easily usable and comprehensive from the viewpoint of any particular subject, an Index and Cross Reference Guide has been added. Here will be listed the exact entries in which appear certain terms for which the reader may look, and also, under key words themselves, other most important entries related to the particular key word. Thus, at a glance, the reader is given a key to comprehensive information surrounding any particular subject. For example, under *hormone* related terms are listed: see also *ACTH, adrenal gland, adrenalin, cortisone, endocrine, gland, ovary, parathyroid, pineal gland, pituitary, testis, testosterone, thymus, thyroid, thyroxin,* etc.

It is the author's sincere hope that this small, simplified dictionary will prove of lasting service to all of those who need to convey medical ideas by way of the written or spoken word and to all who are recipients of such ideas.

H. S.

TABLES AND PLATES

The illustrations of the human skeleton (from Hunter and Hunter, *Biology in Our Lives*) and those of other parts of the body (all from Brownell and Williams, *The Human Body*) are included with the kind permission of the American Book Company. The table of desirable weights is used by courtesy of the Metropolitan Life Insurance Company.

PRONUNCIATION KEY

Fine shades of pronunciation have been eliminated in this dictionary and only the easily apparent differences have been emphasized. For the sake of simplicity, pronunciation has been spelled out as it sounds without the use of symbols. Below are listed the common letter combinations used to indicate sounds.

ay as *a* in *ale, fate*
aa as *a* in *add, ask*
ah as *a* in *bar, far*

ee as *e* in *meet, reed*
eh as *e* in *get, met*

igh as *i* in *sigh, tie*
ih as *i* in *sick, ill*

oh as *o* in *low, no*
aw as *o* in *bought, orb*
oy as *oi* in *oil, goiter*
oo as *oo* in *food, mood*
ow as *ou* in *out, gout*
u as *u* in *dull, cut*
you as *u* in *cute, pure*

zh as *z* in *azure*

th as *th* in *thin, through*

The sign *uh* is used to denote the dull sound that vowels take in unstressed syllables. It does not mean that these sounds should be pronounced absolutely alike in all cases, but only that they are reduced in strength and clarity, as:

a in *among, sofa*
e in *copper, below*
i in *classify, continent*
o in *confer, million*
u in *radium, campus*

A

abasia (*uh-bay'zih-uh*). A condition in which walking is difficult or impossible because of improper or nonfunctioning control of the leg muscles. Thus abasia occurs when a leg "falls asleep" or a "Charley horse" develops. —*astasia a.* Inability to walk or stand due to emotional illness. A symptom of neurosis. —*ataxic a.* Clumsy, unsure walking due to any cause. —*choreic a.* Inability to walk or stand due to spasm of the leg muscles brought on by a nervous condition called *chorea.* —*paralytic a.* Inability of the legs to support the body due to paralysis, as in infantile paralysis, a stroke, or injury to the spinal cord. —*paroxysmal trepidant a.* Cramping and spasm of the legs when walking is attempted. Due to emotional illness, a form of *astasia a.* —*trembling a.* Inability to walk because of marked trembling of the legs.

abdomen. The large body cavity that contains the stomach and intestines, liver, spleen, pancreas, kidneys, and other organs and structures. Commonly called the belly. —*acute a.* Any emergency condition within the belly requiring immediate operation, such as appendicitis, ruptured ulcer, or gunshot wounds of the intestine. —*scaphoid a.* A condition in which the front belly wall is sunken. Seen at times in starvation. Also called *navicular a.*

abduct. Movement of an extremity away from the body, or of a part from the middle of the whole, as the lifting of the arm from the side or the spreading of the fingers.

ablation. Detachment or removal of an organ or part, usually by surgery. The removal of an eye is an example.

abortion. 1. Expulsion of the contents of a pregnant womb to terminate further development of the embryo (or fetus). Used technically when expulsion occurs within the first three months of pregnancy. When it occurs at from three months to the time when life is possible outside the womb (six months), it is called a *miscarriage* or *immature delivery*; from six to nine months (full term), *premature delivery*. 2. The product of the womb expelled before maturity. *—accidental* (or *spontaneous*) *a.* Unexpected emptying of the womb before maturity. *—artificial* (or *induced*) *a.* Intentional termination of pregnancy by means of medicine or surgery before maturity. *—criminal a.* Illegal abortion. Probably the commonest form of medical malpractice, always fraught with great danger to the patient. *—habitual a.* Successive accidental abortions. *—incomplete a.* Contents of the womb partially expelled with some of the birth tissue remaining in the womb. Usually requires surgical intervention to complete. *—inevitable a.* An abortion which has proceeded to the point where it cannot be prevented. *—missed a.* A condition in which death has occurred within the womb but in which the contents are retained for several weeks. *—partial a.* In multiple pregnancy where one of several developing infants is expelled. *—psychiatric a.* An abortion justified by development or exaggeration of a mental condition by the pregnancy. *—therapeutic a.* Termination of a pregnancy that threatens the health or life of the mother. *—threatened a.* A condition in which abortion seems imminent. Treatment may prevent. *—tubal a.* Expulsion of conception products through the Fallopian tubes into the abdominal cavity.

abrasion. An area where the skin or lining tissue of the mouth, eyes, nose, or hollow organs is worn down by scraping or rubbing, as the "skinning" of the knee in a fall.

abscess. A walled-off collection of pus in any part of the body. A common boil is an example. Abscesses are named according to location, as ear abscess, hand abscess; according to how fast they develop and how long they persist, as acute or chronic; according to their cause, as tuberculous abscess; according to their origin, as *primary a.* arising at the seat of infection, or *secondary a.* arising from infection at a remote site.

absorption. The taking in and assimilation of matter, gas, liquid, or solid by the skin, lining tissues, blood, or lymph vessels. When the necessary elements of the digested food in the intestine pass through the wall of the intestine into the blood and lymph, absorption has occurred. When a medication such as a specific hormone is applied in ointment form by rubbing into the skin, the hormone finds its way through the skin into the blood stream by absorption. When oxygen of the air in the lungs finds its way through the lung tissue into the blood, it does so by absorption.

accommodation. The process by which any part or organ of the body adjusts to environment; thus perspiration during heat is the result of the mechanism by which the body maintains a level internal temperature in the face of environmental rises. Used in particular to mean the adaptation of the eye to various distances by changing the convexity of its crystalline lens.

accouchement (*uh-koosh'muhnt*). Childbirth.

acetabulum (*aa-suh-tab'you-luhm*). A cup-shaped hollow in the hip bone where the head of the thigh bone rests.

acetylcholine (*aas-uh-tihl-koh'leen*). A hormone secreted by various parts of the nervous system, especially the parasympathetics. It helps to hurry nervous impulses across nerve junctions of which there are many in the nervous system and also acts upon the minute blood vessels (capillaries), causing them to increase in diameter and porousness.

achalasia. Hollow, muscular organs, such as the stomach, bladder, intestine, normally contract and relax in rhythm when performing their work. When the ability to relax is absent, achalasia results. An example is "knots in the stomach," usually the accompaniment of emotional tension causing contraction of the intestines without relaxation.

Achilles. Certain heel ailments are called by the name of the Greek hero who was vulnerable only in the heel. The tendon which attaches the calf muscle to the heel bone is known as the *Achilles' tendon*.

achlorhydria (*ay-klawr-high'drih-uh*). Normally the stomach manufactures hydrochloric acid as part of its digestive juice. When this acid is absent a condition of achlorhydria (lack of hydrochloric acid) exists, resulting in disturbances of the digestive and nervous systems, as in pernicious anemia.

achylia (*aa-kigh'lih-uh*). The absence of chyle, a milk-white emulsion of fat globules formed in the intestine that finds its way into the lymph. The result of incomplete or faulty handling of fats in the diet. Seen especially in children in a condition known as *coeliac disease* in which there are present foul-smelling fatty stools and general malnutrition. *See also* chyle. —*a. gastrica*. The diminution or absence of digestive juices formed in the stomach. —*a. pancreatica*. Absence of digestive juices ordinarily formed by the pancreas, resulting in symptoms of coeliac disease.

acid-fast. In order to identify certain bacteria, they are stained with aniline dyes. A distinguishing characteristic of some bacteria is that this stain cannot be removed with acid. Such bacteria are designated acid-fast. Among these are the bacteria which cause tuberculosis and leprosy. "Acid-fast" is commonly used to denote the presence of tuberculosis bacteria, as "acid-fast infection" of the lungs.

acid-forming. Used to characterize those foods which, when digested, leave a residue that is acid, such as meats, poultry, fish, cheese, and others.

acidity. 1. Sourness. 2. The amount of acid contained in any substance. —*a. of the stomach*. Sour stomach due to overproduction of acid by the stomach or by the fermentation of certain foods in the stomach. Acidity is usually associated with heartburn, belching, pain, and distress in the upper abdomen.

acidosis. For normal functioning of the body an exquisite balance exists in the blood between free carbon dioxide (CO_2) as carbonic acid and bound carbon dioxide as sodium bicarbonate. Ordinarily this balance exists in such fashion that an increase in one means an increase in the other; thus a specific ratio is maintained. Under certain circumstances, however, there is an absolute increase in the amount of carbonic acid or an absolute decrease in the amount of sodium bicarbonate, resulting in a change in the ratio favoring the carbonic acid. Acidosis, in its more serious forms, is characterized by severe air hunger (gasping breath), coma, and even death. Acidosis may be caused by any condition, such as continued diarrhea and diabetes, in which the body loses sodium bicarbonate and other alkalies, or which results in carbon dioxide retention, as is the case in drowning.

acne. Inflammation of the oil glands of the skin, commonly on the face, back, and chest. At the mouth of the oil gland, a blackhead forms and develops into a pinkish pimple with or without pus. Usually comes on about puberty. Worse in the winter. Cause still unknown.

acneform. Resembling acne.

acromegaly (*aak-roh-mehg'uh-lih*). A condition resulting from the overactivity and overgrowth of certain cells in the pituitary gland. If such overgrowth and overactivity begin early in life, gigantism results. If it begins later, after the bone growth-centers are no longer active, gigantism does not result but typical changes of acromegaly occur as follows: chin enlarges and protrudes; cheekbones and ridge bones of the eyes become thick and heavy; the hands, feet, fingers, and toes become large and thick; internal organs increase in size; scalp becomes ridged and furrowed; backbone deforms and tends to bow forward in the high back; sugar may appear in the urine; severe headache may be experienced; blindness in the outer halves of both fields of vision

may develop. There is no known cure. *See also* HYPERPITUI-
TARISM.

acromion. An extension of the upper, outer part of the shoulder blade that unites with the outer part of the collarbone
to form a protective arch above the head of the arm bone.

acrophobia. Morbid fear of great heights.

ACTH. Abbreviation for adrenocorticotropic hormone, secreted by the anterior lobe of the pituitary gland that
profoundly influences the functioning of the cortex of the
adrenal gland.

actinic. Refers to those rays of sunlight beyond the violet
end of the spectrum which produce chemical change.

actinomycosis (*aak-tih-noh-migh-koh'sihss*). An infectious
disease most often affecting cattle and hogs and, at times,
man; caused by a mold, *actinomyces*. The jaw is most often
affected as the seat of large tumors discharging an oily yellowish pus. Actinomycosis may affect other parts of the
body. The disease in animals is commonly called *lumpy jaw*
or *wooden tongue.*

acute. Any illness is acute which has a sudden beginning,
short course, and severe symptoms, as acute appendicitis,
acute bronchitis.

Addison's disease. The result of impaired function of the
cortex of the adrenal glands, characterized by loss of weight
and emaciation, anemia, progressive darkening of the complexion. Often ends in death.

adduct. Movement of an extremity toward the body, or
parts toward the whole, as the dropping of the arm to the
side, the drawing together of spread fingers, etc.

adenitis (*aad-uh-nigh'tihss*). Inflammation of a gland. An
example is tuberculous adenitis of the neck, an inflammation
of glands in the neck known as scrofula, resulting from infection with tuberculosis germs. Neck glands infected with
tuberculosis become large and break down, discharging pus.

adenoid. 1. Gland-like. 2. Overgrowth of lymph tissue high in the throat behind the nose; appears especially in children. Also called pharyngeal tonsil.

adenoidectomy. Surgical removal of the adenoids.

adenoma (*aad-uh-noh′muh*). A tumor, malignant or benign, which in structure resembles a gland. Classified according to site of origin, as thyroid adenoma.

adenopathy (*aad-uh-nahp′uh-thih*). Any disease of the glands, especially the enlargement of the lymph glands. For example, the enlargement of the neck glands in measles, or the groin glands in venereal disease (*buboes*).

adhesion. The abnormal union of an organ or part to another, e.g. union of lung and pleura, usually caused by inflammation.

adipose. Fatty; fat-like; fat.

adjuvant. 1. A medication which is added to aid the action of another, as phenacetin used with aspirin to increase its effect on fever and pain. 2. An auxiliary, as the drugs used in addition to diet in the treatment of stomach ulcers.

adnexa. The appendages or accessory parts of an organ, as of the eye: the lids, tear glands, and ducts; or of the womb: the Fallopian tubes and ovaries.

adrenal gland. A small gland that lies immediately above each of the two kidneys. The adrenal gland consists of an outer shell, the *cortex*; and an inner core, the *medulla*. These two glands are vital to life, producing different hormones from each of their parts—adrenalin (from the medulla) and corticosterone (from the cortex), from which, among other compounds, cortisone is made. (Cortisone may also be synthetically produced.)

adrenalin. Also called epinephrine. The most important hormone secreted by the core or medulla of the adrenal glands. It acts principally to contract the small blood vessels, to stimulate the heart, and to relax the bronchial tubes. Adrenalin plays a special part in the sugar metabolism taking place in the liver. Whereas insulin helps to store sugar in the liver in the form of glycogen, adrenalin restores the sugar for use as the body's main fuel for producing energy.

adventitious (*aad-vuhn-tih'shuhss*). 1. Accidental or acquired as differentiated from usual or natural. 2. Pertaining to the *adventitia*, the tough outer coat of an organ or blood vessel. 3. Occurring in unusual places. For example, adventitious sounds of the heart are: the murmurs of various diseases, as rheumatic fever; of the lungs: the raspings, wheezings, bubblings, musical notes heard in the course of diseases such as pneumonia, asthma, and tumors.

afebrile (*aa-fee'bruhl*). Without fever.

affect. Feeling; mood; emotion.

afterbirth. The membranes and organized tissue expelled from the womb following childbirth.

agar (*aa'guhr*). 1. A seaweed. 2. An easily melted solid made from seaweed and used in the laboratory as a medium for the growth of bacteria. —*a. agar*. A mucilaginous extract of agar commonly used as a laxative; when in the intestine it absorbs moisture, swells considerably, and thus stimulates intestinal movement and evacuation.

agitation. 1. Restlessness with violent motion. 2. Mental illness.

agnosia. Total or partial loss of the faculty by which persons or things are recognized. Commonly designated according to the sense involved. —*auditory a.* Hearing but not understanding what is said. —*optic a.* Seeing but not recognizing; —*tactile a.* Sense of touch is not impaired but there is no recognition of the object touched.

agony. 1. The death struggle at the end of disease or injury. 2. Extreme anguish, severe pain.

agoraphobia. A morbid fear of open places or spaces.

agranulocytosis (*aa-graan-you-loh-sigh-toh'sihss*). A disease of sudden onset, high fever, prostration with ulcerations in the mouth, throat, and elsewhere. In the blood there is a marked decrease in the number of white cells that have granules in their protoplasm. May be fatal. Usually induced by an allergy to certain drugs.

ague (*ay'gyou*). Repeated chills. Formerly used to designate an attack of malaria.

air sickness. *See* MOTION SICKNESS.

airway. One of a number of instruments used to keep the breathing passages clear during the use of a general anesthetic.

ala. Any wing-like part. —*a. nasi.* The flared outer part of the nostril. —*a. auris.* The outer ear.

alalia (*aa-lay'lih-uh*). Loss or impairment of speech, usually caused by a physical defect.

albumen. A protein, the most important constituent of animal tissues. Classified according to source as *muscle a., egg a., serum a.*

albuminuria. The presence of albumen and other proteins in the urine. The normal kidney does not permit these blood elements to pass through. When the kidney is diseased these elements may find their way into the urine. Their presence is at times accounted for by pus or blood from the kidney itself. This finding is present in a great variety of conditions, including heart disease, nutritional deficiencies, fevers, brain injury, gout, goiter, apoplexy, and others.

alcoholism. 1. Poisoning with alcohol. 2. The physical and mental condition that results from excessive or prolonged use of intoxicating drinks. —*acute a.* Drunkenness; inebriety. —*chronic a.* The state caused by prolonged and repeated excesses of alcoholic indulgences accompanied by severe digestive and nervous disturbances.

algesia (*aal-jee'zih-uh*). Sensitivity to pain.

alienist. A psychiatrist, especially one who testifies in insanity hearings.

alimentary. 1. Pertaining to act of nutrition. 2. Related to food and nutrition. 3. Related to or produced by diet. —*a. tract* or *a. canal.* The digestive tube from the mouth to the anus including the gullet, stomach, and intestine.

alimentation. The act of nutrition.

alkalosis. *See* ACIDOSIS, of which this is the opposite. Alkalosis results when, under unusual circumstances, the balance of the blood is disturbed by an increase in the amount of sodium bicarbonate. This disturbance is characterized by a very slow pulse, dizziness, and uncontrollable jerky movements of the muscles. If not corrected it may be fatal. Common causes are persistent vomiting in which the stomach acid ordinarily used to produce carbonic acid never reaches the blood because it is expelled with the vomitus, forced breathing in which carbon dioxide is expelled in large amounts, and the intake of large amounts of sodium bicarbonate.

allergen (*aal'luhr-jehn*). Any agent capable of producing an allergic reaction; usually refers to material agents, as pollen, animal hairs, fungi, foods, worms, bacteria, drugs.

allergist. A physician who specializes in allergic diseases.

allergy. A state of unusual sensitivity to various elements of the environment. This sensitivity represents an overreaction of the individual to one or many aspects of the environment or to products of his own body. Generally there are two major types of allergy: *acquired*, as sensitivity to penicillin; *hereditary*, as sensitivity to food or pollen. Any aspect of the environment may cause allergic reactions. Allergens are generally *material*, as foods, bacteria, pollen, animal hairs; *physical*, heat, cold, light; *emotional*, feelings, moods, personality patterns which have their roots in childhood. Examples of allergic diseases are hay fever, asthma, hives, eczema, drug reactions, serum sickness, poison ivy, and others.

alogia (*ay-loh'jih-uh*). 1. The inability to speak due to an injury in that part of the brain that controls the use of language. 2. Stupid or senseless behavior.

alopecia (*aa-loh-pee'shuh*). Baldness.

altitude sickness. The symptoms resulting from the lower amount of oxygen in the air at high altitudes in airplane flights. —*acute a.s.* May result from a single flight in headache, more effortful breathing, general distress, anxiety, weakness, fatigue, sleepiness, depression, or an unusual sense of well-being. —*chronic a.s.* Follows repeated flights at high altitude. Symptoms are headache, fatigue, irritability, nervousness, sleeplessness, increased appetite, inability to concentrate, lack of will; at times nausea, indigestion, dizziness, lack of appetite.

amaurosis. (*aam-aw-roh'sihss*). Partial or total blindness.

amblyopia. Dimness of vision which does not result from actual disease of the eye itself or from errors of refraction. Often due to disease of the optic nerve or brain. During prohibition alcoholic amblyopia was common.

amenorrhea (*aa-mehn-uh-ree'uh*). Absence of menstruation due to pregnancy or disease.

amino acid. When proteins are broken down by the digestive processes, the final products are amino acids, which the body stores for use as needed to rebuild protein and to manufacture other necessary compounds. There are 22 known amino acids; ten are considered essential to life.

amorphous. 1. Shapeless; without form. 2. In biology, lack of structure. 3. In chemistry, not crystalline. Examples: sulphur powder is amorphous; at conception, the fertilized egg is amorphous.

ampule (ampul, ampoule). A container, ordinarily made of glass, capable of being sealed hermetically and used to hold sterile medication for injection.

ampulla. The widened end of a small passageway, such as the tear duct, the milk duct.

amyotonia (*aa-migh-oh-toh'nih-uh*). The absence or marked decrease of the normal state of tension of muscles; flaccidity of muscles. —*a. congenita.* Also called *Oppenheim's disease,* a disease occurring at birth which involves the spinal cord and stem of the brain. Mental development is normal but there is marked impairment of the ability to sit up, stand, or walk.

anabolism. The conversion of food into more complex living matter. The constructive aspect of metabolism, as the use of the simple amino acids by the body to build up highly complex proteins in replacement of worn-out tissues.

anal erotism (*ay'nuhl ehr'uh-tihsm*). Sensations of pleasure derived from the act of defecation or other stimulation of the anus. Experienced particularly in childhood and ordinarily repressed later.

analgesia. Insensibility to pain without the loss of consciousness. —*continuous caudal a.* A method by which the pain of childbirth is relieved by a continuous flow of anesthetic solution low in the spinal canal. —*infiltration a.* Injection of an anesthetic under the skin or other tissue to paralyze the nerve endings at the site of operation.

analgesic. Any agent which relieves pain.

analysand. One undergoing psychoanalysis.

anemia. A condition commonly called "thin blood," in which the normal blood manufacturing processes are inadequate. May be caused by a loss of the total amount of blood, as after serious bleeding; a reduction in the number of red blood cells; a reduction in the amount of material contained within the red blood cells (hemoglobin), or both. The condition is characterized by breathlessness, dizziness, palpitation of the heart, lack of skin color, weakness. —*deficiency a.* Caused by inadequate diet. —*hemolytic a.* Caused by any agent that destroys red blood cells, as cobra venom. —*hemorrhagic a.* Caused by copious bleeding. —*macrocytic a.* Characterized by larger than normal red blood cells with little hemoglobin. Found in pernicious anemia, sprue, and anemia of pregnancy. —*pernicious a.* A condition in which the red blood cells do not grow to maturity. Maturing of red blood cells depends upon a substance manufactured in the lining tissue of the lower end of the stomach and the small intestine and also upon certain substances that come from food. —*plastic a.* A serious condition, often fatal, resulting from a defect of the bone marrow which is the organ of red blood cell formation. Here, both the number of red blood cells and amount of hemoglobin are seriously reduced. In addition, there is a decrease in the number of certain necessary white blood cells.

anesthesia. Loss of sensation. May be intentional, through the use of various agents as before an operation, or the result of one of a great number of diseases. The latter type is named according to the site of, or disease causing, anesthesia.

anesthesiology. The specialty devoted to the study and administration of local and general anesthetics.

anesthetic. A drug which produces a loss of sensibility, local or general.

aneurysm (*aan'yuh-rihsm*). The weakening and stretching of part of the wall of an artery, or the heart, that may result in the formation of a sac at the weak point, much like the ballooning out of a weak spot in an inner tube or a water hose. Aneurysm, the sac or ballooned-out portion, is often associated with pain and symptoms of pressure. These vary in seriousness with the location of the aneurysm in the body. Thus, if the aneurysm is in an artery near one of the large nerves of the arm, it may cause pain, loss of sensation, and/or paralysis of the arm. Most commonly it occurs in the major artery leading from the heart, the aorta, often as a result of syphilis, although other diseases may produce it.

angina (*aan-jigh'nuh*). 1. Any disease characterized by attacks of suffocation, especially an involvement of the tonsil area or throat. 2. Sore throat. 3. Cramplike pain or spasms. —*a. pectoris.* Considered a psychosomatic condition and characterized by severe pressure and heaviness in the chest. Pain shoots from the heart region to the left shoulder, then down the arm into the fingers, and is accompanied by a sense of impending death. Chiefly affects men over forty and is rare in women. —*agranulocytic a.* Severe choking pain in the throat associated with the condition known as *agranulocytosis.*

ankylosis. The stiffening of a joint by disease or operation; the stiffness of a joint the bones of which are firmly united or bound down by adhesions, as the permanent stiffness of the ankle joint resulting from a bad break and inadequate treatment.

annulus (*aan'yuh-luhss*). A ring-shaped or circular opening. Examples are the mouth, the upper and lower ends of the stomach, the anus.

anodyne. Medicine that relieves pain, as aspirin or codein.

anomaly. An abnormality; any deviation from the usual; any part or organ or system existing in an abnormal form, location, or construction. Thus *dextrocardia* (the heart on the right side), *polydactylism* (more than five fingers), and *albinism* (lack of pigment) are anomalies.

anopsia. Disuse of vision; for instance, if, due to defective eye muscles, the eyes are turned upward permanently so that the individual is prevented from using them for vision; or if vision is interfered with by factors of psychological origin, as sometimes in hysteria.

anorchism. Absence of testes, as in the eunuch.

anorexia. Absence of appetite.

anoscope. A tubular instrument inserted into the rectum for visual examination of its interior.

anosmia. Absence of the sense of smell.

anoxemia. A reduction in the normal amount of oxygen in the blood when insufficient air reaches the blood. Due often to high altitude, or to low oxygen content of inhaled gas, as in anesthesia, heart failure, strangling.

anoxia. An insufficient supply of oxygen and the body disturbances that result. —*anemic a.* Caused by the reduction of the ability of the blood to carry oxygen, as in anemias where the oxygen carrier, hemoglobin, is reduced in amount. —*anoxic a.* Due to an interference in the normal penetrability of the lungs by oxygen, so that oxygen does not get into the blood. Results from various lung diseases and is the technical cause of drowning. —*histotoxic a.* Arises from an inability of the body cells to use the oxygen which penetrates the lung in normal amount and is adequately carried by a normal amount of hemoglobin. Disturbance of normal function of body cells is produced by various poisons, including alcohol and narcotics. —*stagnant a.* Where penetrability of the lungs by oxygen, carriage of oxygen by the hemoglobin in the blood, utilization of oxygen by the cells are normal, but the speed of the flow of blood is reduced, and the body cells do not receive enough oxygen. This condition can be *general*, taking place all over the body at the same time, as in collapse or shock; or it may be *local* in one organ or area of an organ as the result of spasm or blockage of an artery.

antabuse. A drug for the treatment of alcoholism.

antacid. A substance that relieves acidity or neutralizes acids, as bicarbonate of soda or milk.

antemortem. Before death.

antenatal. Before birth; occurring or existing before birth.

ante-partum. Before maternal delivery.

anterior. Situated in front of, or before; the forward part of an organ. Examples: the belly wall is an anterior structure; the face is on the anterior aspect of the body.

anteversion. The forward displacement, tipping, or tilting of an organ or part, especially the womb.

anthelmintic (*aan-thehl-mihn'tihk*). Destructive of worms. Ordinarily refers to drugs whose purpose it is to rid the intestinal tract of worms.

anthracosis. Blackening of the lungs associated with a mild, long-standing inflammation. Arises from the prolonged inhalation of carbon dust, frequently found among coal miners.

anthrax. An infectious disease of sheep and cattle that may be transmitted to man. Caused by a germ, *bacillus anthracis*.— Also called *woolsorter's disease, tanner's disease, splenic fever, ragpicker's disease, malignant pustule.*

antianemic principle. A substance that prevents or counteracts anemia, found in the liver and used most often in the treatment of pernicious anemia.

antiarthritic. 1. A remedy for arthritis. 2. Tending to relieve or cure arthritis.

antibiotic. An extract made of certain micro-organisms that is employed against infections caused by other organisms, as penicillin, aureomycin, terramycin, streptomycin, chloromycetin.

antibody. A class of protective substances found in the body naturally, or produced in the body by the stimulating action of another class of substances known as *antigens*. Antigens are mostly protein in nature and may be parts of living organisms such as bacteria. Thus, the virus of measles when it enters the body stimulates the production of antibodies of measles which protect the afflicted individual from further encroachment by the virus during the initial disease and from future susceptibility to the disease.

antidote. Anything that neutralizes or prevents the action of a poison.

antigen (*aan'tih-jehn*). A protein or protein-linked substance that is capable of stimulating the body to produce antibodies, as disease germs, tetanus injections. *See also* ANTIBODY.

antipyretic. Anything that reduces fever. The most important antipyretics are cold, perspiration producers, quinine, and many of the coal-tar drugs, as aspirin, acetanilide, and antipyrine.

antisepsis. The prevention of contamination with germs by stopping their growth or multiplication, in contradistinction to disinfection where the germs are actually killed.

antitoxin. A specific antibody capable of neutralizing or checking a specific toxin or poison from plant, animal, or bacteria. Example: tetanus antitoxin, an antitoxin that specifically inactivates the poison produced by the tetanus or lockjaw germ.

antrum. 1. A hollow space, especially in a bone. 2. The sinuses in the face under the eyes, also called *maxillary sinuses*.

anuria. The suppression of urine.

anus (*ay'nuhss*). The outlet of the digestive tract; the terminal portion of the rectum.

aorta. The largest artery in the body that rises directly from the heart, branches in many directions, and is thus eventually responsible for the distribution of blood to all parts of the body.

aortitis (*ay-awr-tigh'tihss*). Inflammation of the aorta. Aortitis may result from a number of diseases, as rheumatic fever and syphilis.

aperient. A mild purgative or laxative, as milk of magnesia, Castoria.

aphagia (*uh-fay'jih-uh*). Loss of the ability to swallow.

aphakia. The normal eye has a lens situated behind the pupil. Where this lens is absent, aphakia exists. May be a defect at birth or the result of surgery or injury.

aphasia. An impairment of the capacity to use words as symbols of ideas, following an injury in the higher centers of the brain that control this complex association function. People with this condition may speak an unintelligible jargon or repeat over and over certain phrases or words, although there is no reason to believe they do not formulate ideas. Aphasia does not refer to a defect in the mechanics of hearing or speaking, but only to a disturbance in the use of language for the conveyance of thought. There are many degrees and forms of aphasia depending upon the area of the brain diseased or injured. Aphasia is often seen after a stroke or blood clot on the brain.

aphonia. Loss of the power of speech.

aphrodisiac. Any agent stimulating the sexual desire.

apoplexy. A "stroke," often resulting in one-sided paralysis, coma, and death. Ordinarily due to an injury to, or closure of, a vital blood vessel of the brain.

appendectomy. The surgical removal of the appendix.

applicator. Any instrument used to make local applications of medicine or treatment of any sort, as the medicated cotton swab inserted into the nose, the plate of a diathermy machine.

apraxia. A condition characterized by inability to make

purposeful movements although there is no evidence of paralysis or loss of sensation. The difficulty lies in the higher centers of the brain that control the translation of the desire or need to make a movement, and the muscular action required for such a movement.

arachnidism. (*uh-raak'nih-dihsm*). A condition that results from the bite of a poisonous spider.

arachnoid (*uh-raak'noyd*). A very fine, thin tissue, as the middle of the three layers that cover the brain and spinal cord.

areola. (*aa-ree'uh-lah*). A ring of color surrounding a particular point or space, as the nipple or a small boil. —*a. mammae.* The colored area that surrounds the nipples of the breasts. During pregnancy this area becomes much larger, producing a distinct second ring of color surrounding the first. —*umbilical a.* A colored ring that surrounds the navel in some people.

argyria (*ahr-jigh'rih-uh*). A dark or bluish-gray discoloration of the skin and/or lining tissues of the mouth, nose, eyes, and intestinal tract produced by prolonged use of various silver preparations as medicine or as occupational material. The discoloration results from the gradual deposition of small granules of silver in the tissues.

ariboflavinosis. Deficiency of riboflavin, one of the main parts of the vitamin-B complex, characterized by inflammation, cracking and small sores of the lips and the clear part of the eye; also an oily inflammation of the skin.

armamentarium. All of the instruments, the laboratory and treatment equipment, the medicines, the journals, the books used by a physician to assist him in the practice of his profession.

arrest. A stopping, restraining, or checking. —*cardiac a.* A standstill of the entire heart, cessation of the heartbeat. —*pelvic a.* A condition in maternal labor in which part of the developing infant becomes fixed in a certain position in the bony framework of the mother's pelvis. —*transverse a.* A condition resulting from a type of flat, maternal pelvis which causes the head of the developing infant to be fixed in a horizontal position.

arrhythmia. A disturbance of normal rhythm, as in the heartbeat or pulse.

arsenical. A drug that depends for its effect upon its arsenic content. Commonly employed in the treatment of syphilis.

arteriole. The smallest sized artery.

arterioplasty. An operation, usually for aneurysm, in which the artery is reconstructed by using the walls of the aneurysm to restore the blood vessel's continuity.

arteriosclerosis. Hardening of the arteries produced by an increase in fibrous tissue within the walls of the artery. Fat and calcium are also accumulated within the artery walls, which results in a loss of elasticity of the blood vessel and therefore a loss of its ability to contract. The cause is not known.

arteritis. Inflammation of an artery.

artery. One of the two major types of blood vessel characterized primarily by carrying blood *from* the heart *to* other parts of the body. Its wall is ordinarily composed of three coats of tissue: an *outer* coat, elastic and fibrous; a *middle* coat, elastic and muscular; and an *inner* coat, very similar to the lining membrane of other hollow organs, such as the intestine and mouth.

arthralgia (*ahr-thraal'jih-uh*). Pain in a joint.

arthritis. Inflammation of a joint. There are numerous types classified according to severity, location, deformity, cause.

arthrodesis (*ahr-throh-dee'sihss*). Permanent stiffening of a joint, as the knee, by surgical removal of the cartilage (gristle) which lines the ends of the bone and permits movement.

arthroplasty. 1. Surgically rebuilding a stiffened joint into a normally functioning one. 2. Any operation upon a joint to make it function.

articulation. 1. Enunciation of speech. 2. A joint; the meeting or junction of two or more bones.

asbestosis. A condition of the lungs resulting from prolonged inhalation of dust containing asbestos.

ascariasis (*aas-kuh-righ'uh-sihss*). An invasion of the body
by roundworms. The areas most commonly involved are the
intestine, stomach, liver, and lungs.

ascites (*uh-sigh'teez*). An abnormal accumulation of fluid
in the abdominal cavity, characterized by painless enlargement of the abdomen. Ascites is most frequently associated
with heart failure, certain liver diseases, kidney failure.
Dropsy is an archaic word for this condition.

ascorbic acid. The chemical name for vitamin C; also called
cevitamic acid, anti-scorbutic vitamin, and *avitamic acid.* It
is essential for life and is especially important in wound
healing and tissue repair. It is found in fresh green foods,
citrus fruits, and other uncooked foods. An absolute lack of
this acid leads to *scurvy*.

asepsis. The exclusion of bacteria which produce decay.

aspergillosis (*aas-puhr-jihl-loh'sihss*). Infection with a type
of fungus known as *aspergillus*. Any part of the body may
be involved, especially the lungs, bronchial tubes, outer ear,
sinuses, bones, or coverings of the brain.

aspermatism. Defective or absent semen; the nonformation
of sperm.

asphyxia. Suffocation; unconsciousness that results from the
deprivation of oxygen.

aspirator. An apparatus used to withdraw liquids from body
cavities, as in the sucking out of pus from sinuses.

asthenia. The absence or loss of strength that occurs in the
course of certain diseases such as tuberculosis, in malnutrition, and in certain emotional states.

asthma. Usually refers to allergic asthma characterized by
attacks of shortness of breath, coughing, wheezing, a thick
phlegm, and a sense of oppression or constriction in the
chest. Caused by allergy to things eaten, breathed, touched,
or to bacteria that live in various body cavities, such as the

sinuses or gall bladder, or in various organs or parts such as the teeth and tonsils.

astigmatism. Faulty vision that results from an irregularity in the curvature of one or more of the surfaces of the eye that ordinarily permit light to pass straight through. Astigmatism may occur at birth or later in life. There are many varieties classified according to how the light is distorted in passing through the eye curvature; that is, whether the distortion is vertical, horizontal, oblique.

atherosclerosis. A form of hardening of the arteries, the result of accumulation of fat in the *inner wall* of the arteries.

athetosis. A condition usually affecting children, characterized by constant, uncontrollable, slow motion of the fingers, toes, hands, feet and other parts of the body. Ordinarily the result of injury to or disease of the brain.

athlete's foot. *See* epidermophytosis, dermophytosis.

atlas. The topmost vertebra in the spinal column.

atomization. The breaking up of a liquid into a fine spray, as in liquid medicines used for spraying the nose and throat.

atony. A low degree or absence of tone, as of a muscle. Lack of normal tension. Flaccidity. Example: atony of the bladder, the inability of the bladder to expel urine because of inefficient muscular power.

atopy. The familial or hereditary type of allergy, as distinguished from the acquired form. Examples are hay fever, eczema, asthma.

atresia. The absence or permanent closure of a normally occurring opening or canal, as atresia of the vagina, anus, ear canal, pupil.

atrophy (*aat'ruh-fih*). The reduction in size of an organ or cell that previously had reached mature size. This reduction may be normal or abnormal. Example of the normal is shrinkage of tonsils or thymus gland with age. Example of the abnormal is shrinkage and wasting of muscles when not in use because of disease.

attenuation. A weakening, thinning, or diluting; especially a reduction in the poisonous quality of a virus or other micro-organism.

audiogram. A graphic record showing the hearing ability of an individual as indicated by a machine called an *audiometer*.

audiology. The science of hearing.

audiometer. An instrument for measuring the range of acuteness of hearing.

auditory. Relating to the act or organs of hearing.

aura. One or a group of sensations experienced as premonitions of the onset of an attack of a particular disease. For example; in epilepsy, asthma, or migraine, patients may experience strange odors, flashes of light, itching between the shoulder blades, or other sensations warning of the imminence of an attack.

aural. Pertaining to the ear or to hearing.

aureomycin. An antibiotic produced by, and derived from, a fungus known as *streptomyces*.

aurotherapy. Treatment with gold salts for arthritis and various skin diseases. Gold salts in liquid form are given by injection into a vein.

auscultation (*aw-skuhl-tay'shuhn*). A method of diagnosis by the study and detection of sound arising from various organs, particularly the heart and lungs. When the physician uses his stethoscope he is employing auscultation to help in diagnosis.

Australian X disease. An epidemic virus disease which produces inflammation of the brain. The disease resembles infantile paralysis. It is very common in children and first appeared in Australia in 1917.

autism. Morbid concentration, an exclusive interest in fantasy and daydreaming.

autoanamnesis (*aw-tuh-aan-aam-nee'sihss*). The history of a patient's condition related by himself.

autoclave. 1. *n.* An apparatus used for the sterilization of objects by steam heat under high pressure. 2. *v.* To sterilize in an autoclave.

autodigestion. Literally "to digest itself," as the digestion of the walls of the stomach by stomach juice when disease of the stomach is present, as in the formation of an ulcer.

autoerotism. Sexual stimulation of self without resort to another person.

autogenous (*aw-tahj'uh-nuhss*). Self-generated. Arising within the organism itself, as applied to various diseases, as diabetes or hardening of the arteries; to toxins, and to especially prepared vaccines. An example of autogenous vaccine is one made from the excretions of the individual, as of the pus in his sinuses, and used in his treatment.

autointoxication. Poisoning by products elaborated within the body through faulty metabolism. At one time this poisoning was thought to occur from severe constipation.

autolysis (*aw-tahl'ih-sihss*). The self-digestion of tissues within the living body. For example, the destructive action in some instances of the blood serum of an animal or a human upon its own red blood cells.

autonomic. Self-governing; independent in action or function. Applied particularly to a special nervous system that operates exclusive of will.

autopsy. An examination of the body after death to discover the actual cause of death.

autotransfusion. 1. The forcing of blood into vital areas after unusual hemorrhage or in order to prevent the onset of shock, performed by elevating three of the extremities and applying constricting bandages to them. By not permitting the blood to enter the extremities, it is forced to remain in the vital areas. 2. Reintroduction by injection into a vein of the blood or serum lost during an operation, especially in the abdominal cavity.

avitamic acid. Vitamin C or ascorbic acid.

avitaminosis. Any disease which results from a deficiency of vitamins.

avulsion. A tearing or wrenching away of a part. —*a. of bulb.* Forcible separation of the eyeball from its socket through tearing of the muscles, tendons, and optic nerve.

axilla. The armpit.

Ayerza's syndrome (*ay-yuhr'zahs*). A disease described by the Argentine physician Abel Ayerza. Characterized by bluish discoloration of the skin and lips, breathlessness, and hardening of the major artery of the lung. Dr. Ayerza thought this to be an independent condition. Today it is known to be produced by syphilis, rheumatic disease of the heart, increase of pressure in the blood that circulates through the lungs, and hardening of the arteries that lead the blood into the lungs.

azoospermia (*ay-zoh-oh-spuhr'mih-uh*). An absence of sperm in the semen.

B

bacillary. Relating to a certain type of rod-shaped bacteria known as *bacillus.*

bacillemia. The presence of bacilli in the blood.

bacilluria. The presence of bacilli in the urine.

bacillus *pl.* bacilli. One of three major forms of bacteria. A rod-shaped organism that may be slender and short, straight or slightly bent. Many types of bacilli exist; examples are leprosy b., tuberculosis b.

bacitracin (*baas'ih-tray-sihn*). An antibiotic obtained from the *bacillus subtilis.*

back. The posterior part of the trunk from the neck to the pelvic girdle.

bacteremia. Presence of bacteria in the blood.

bacteria, *sing.* bacterium. An extremely large group of microscopic single-celled organisms, vegetable in nature, that exist as ovals or spheres (*cocci*), rods (*bacilli*), spirals (*spirilla*), and a small group of comma-shaped organisms (*vibrios*). The cocci may appear in pairs (*diplococci*), or in chains (*streptococci*), or in clusters (*staphylococci*). A small part of this very large group of organisms, commonly called germs, may cause disease among animals and humans. Most of them, however, do not.

bactericide. Any agent or condition that destroys bacteria.

bacteriophage (*baak-tih'rih-uh-fayj*). An agent that produces the dissolution of certain bacteria. Bacteriophage is too small to be seen through the ordinary microscope, but can be transmitted from one bacterial culture to another. The agent may be a living organism, like a virus, or it may be an enzyme.

bacteriostasis (*baak-tih-rih-uh-stay'sihss*). Stopping or hindering the growth of bacteria.

bacteriuria (*baak-tih-rih-you'rih-uh*). The presence of bacteria in the urine.

bagassosis. A lung disease that occurs in workmen who handle the dry residue bagasse in sugar cane after the juice has been extracted. The disease comes on suddenly and its symptoms are difficulty in breathing, fever, coughing. On X-ray, the lungs show a fine mottling and the presence of small fibers of sugar cane.

BAL (*baal*). A chemical developed during World War II, highly effective against lewisite, a poison gas. Also a potent antidote for other arsenical gases, against arsenic in overdoses when used in the treatment of syphilis, and in mercury and other metallic-salt poisonings. Given by injection into muscle.

balanatis (*baal-uh-nigh'tihss*). An inflammation of the tip of the penis or of the clitoris.

balanus (*baal'uh-nuhss*). The glans (tip) of the penis or of the clitoris.

baldness. *See* alopecia, calvities.

Balkan frame. A frame of four supports attached to the bed-posts several feet above the level of the bed and used to suspend broken limbs by means of splints so that continuous traction by weights and pulleys is possible.

ballistocardiograph. An instrument used to record the various movements of the body caused by the impact and recoil of the blood after it is expressed from the heart. The instrument estimates the blood output of the heart and the record that results is called a *ballistocardiogram.*

ballottement (*buh-laht'muhnt*). The bouncing back or rebound of a part when pressure upon it is released. Important procedure in the diagnosis of a number of conditions, as in "water on the knee" where the examiner can push the knee cap back and when he releases this pressure, the knee cap bounds forward to its former position.

barbiturism. A state of intoxication or poisoning following an overdose of barbiturate drugs, such as seconal, nembutal, phenobarbital. The symptoms are tremors, loss of muscular co-ordination, mental confusion, occasional skin eruptions, delirium, coma, and at times death.

barium sulfate. A white, tasteless, odorless powder used in an emulsion that the patient drinks when X-rays of the stomach and intestines are made. Barium sulfate does not permit the passage of X-rays, thus producing a shadow of the passageway through the gastrointestinal tract.

Bartholinitis. Inflammation of the Bartholin glands situated in the forward part of the vagina.

basal metabolic rate. The amount of energy expended by the individual, per unit of time, under resting conditions. *See also* METABOLISM.

basilic vein. The large vein often seen on the inner side of the upper arm.

BCG. Usually indicates a vaccine prepared from an organism known as bacillus Calmette-Guerin. This vaccine is made from a weakened strain of tuberculosis bacilli and is employed in some parts of the world for immunization against tuberculosis.

bearing down. In certain diseases the feeling of weight or pressure in the lower abdomen or pelvis. —*b.d. pains.* The pains experienced in labor that are premonitory of, and accompany, expulsion of the fetus.

bed sore. An ulcer of the skin caused by pressure against the bed. One of the dangers of confining illnesses.

bends. A condition caused by a too rapid return from high air pressure to normal pressure. Suffered by tunnel workers, sand hogs, divers, and others who work under high atmospheric pressure. Bends is due to the formation of nitrogen bubbles in the blood, just as bubbles appear in carbonated water when it is poured or squirted from the bottle. Symptoms depend upon the location of the bubbles and may be as follows: pain, numbness, tingling, paralyses, itching, choking, unconsciousness. Prompt recovery follows proper treatment. Also called *caisson disease, diver's neurosis, compressed-air illness.*

benign. Innocent; not threatening to health or life; not malignant. Examples: a benign tumor, a benign disease.

beriberi. A disease caused by a lack of one of the vitamins of the B-complex *thiamine.* A variety of symptoms may appear, depending upon the severity and the duration of the vitamin deficiency. Among these symptoms are weakness, paralysis, inflammation of nerves, swelling of the legs, abdomen and chest, mental deterioration, and finally heart failure. Beriberi is particularly common among those who live on a polished rice diet.

beryllosis. An inflammation of the lungs resulting from inhalation of beryllium oxide dust. An occupational disease in those industries using beryllium (the manufacture of fluorescent lamps and the hardening of steel).

biceps. 1. A muscle having two heads. 2. The major muscle of the upper arm.

bile. A green to golden brown liquid alkali produced by the liver and poured into the small intestine. Excess bile is stored in the gall bladder. Of exceedingly bitter taste, its function is to aid in the digestion and absorption of fats, the neutralization of acid from the stomach that finds its way into the intestine, and the prevention of putrefaction in the intestine.

bilharziasis. *See* SCHISTOSOMIASIS.

biliary (*bihl'ih-ehr-ih*). Referring to bile or to the conveying of bile from one part to another, as a biliary duct.

biliousness. A popular term for a condition marked by general weakness, headache, loss of appetite, indigestion, constipation, coated tongue. Biliousness is due to a digestive disorder, but is commonly attributed to excessive bile production.

biliuria. The presence of bile in the urine.

biologicals. Complex medical preparations, such as blood plasma, antitoxins, serums, used in the treatment or prevention of disease by injection.

biopsy. Most commonly refers to the removal of a small bit of tissue for microscopic examination to aid in diagnosis. For example, a small piece of tissue removed from an area suspected of being cancerous for examination under the microscope.

birth injury. Any injury suffered by an infant during the process of being born, such as the break or dislocation of a bone, or various damages to the brain.

birthmark. A mole (mark) of various dimensions that may be colored or uncolored. It may or may not contain an unusual number of blood vessels.

bismuthosis (*bihz-muhth-oh'sihss*). Poisoning following prolonged use of bismuth, a drug commonly used in the treatment of syphilis.

bistoury (*bihss'tuh-rih*). A narrow, long knife, sharp-pointed, straight or curved, used in opening abscesses or severing adhesions.

blackwater fever. A form of malaria in which blood appears in the urine. Usually fatal.

blast injury. Injury resulting from the detonation of high explosives at short range. —*atmospheric b.i.* Injuries resulting when the explosion is in the air or on the earth. The severe pressure on the body causes rupture of small blood vessels in the lungs and is followed by spitting up of blood. Breathlessness, and a bluish discoloration of the skin appear, pneumonia may develop, and shock is profound. Not uncommonly the eardrums are ruptured. —*immersion b.i.* Injuries resulting where the explosion occurs underwater. The organs in the abdominal cavity are most often injured due to the great pressure exerted on the body. The symptoms vary with the organ or parts most affected.

blastomycosis. Any of a variety of diseases caused by a great number of yeast-like fungi. Practically any system and part of the body may be involved, such as the skin, lungs, abdominal organs, bones, brain.

bleb. A blister of the skin or the lining tissues that is filled with serum or blood. An example is the early small blisters of chicken pox.

bleeding disease. *See* HEMOPHILIA.

bleeding time. The time required for the natural stoppage of bleeding from a deep cut in the skin. Ordinarily one to three minutes are required. A knowledge of bleeding time is necessary in diagnosis of certain diseases and before performing operations. Prolongation indicates a defect in the clotting mechanism of the blood.

blepharitis (*blehf-uh-righ'tihss*). Inflammation of the eyelids. There are many and varied types named according to the area of the eyelids involved or the cause of the inflammation.

blepharon. The eyelid.

blister. A small raised area of fluid within the layers of the skin. Blisters are named according to cause, site, contents, and whether or not they shift from one site to another.

blood count. A procedure that determines the number of red and white blood cells per cubic millimeter of blood. An instrument called a *hemocytometer* is used. The tip of the finger or the earlobe is pricked. A drop of blood then is sucked up into a small graduated pipette in exact measure, diluted with the proper fluid, mixed, and examined under the microscope for counting. —*differential b.c.* Ordinarily refers to the estimation of the percentage of each different type of white blood cell per cubic millimeter of blood.

blood pressure. The pressure exerted by the blood upon the walls of the arteries. This pressure depends upon the force of the heartbeat, the total amount and thickness of the blood, the elastic quality of the artery walls, and the resistance offered to the passage of the blood by the smallest caliber blood vessels, the capillaries. Blood pressure is expressed in two figures: the larger one, *systolic,* is the reading obtained at the moment when the heart contracts; and the small one, *diastolic,* is the reading at the time the heart relaxes. The more significant of the two is the diastolic, since it represents the constant smallest load on the heart. The difference between the figures representing systolic and diastolic pressure is called the *pulse pressure* and represents the swing between the active and resting phases of heart action.

blood substitute. When for some reason blood itself cannot be used in transfusion, one of a number of substances or combinations of substances are employed. A few of these are gelatin, acacia, albumin, plasma, solutions of mineral salts.

blood typing. Every individual belongs to one of four major blood types by virtue of certain elements in his blood serum and cells. The process of determining which type is specific to the individual is known as blood typing. This is a most important process since various blood types are incompatible with each other, and transfusing such incompatible blood may result in grave symptoms or death.

bolus. Ordinarily refers to the rounded mass of food prepared for swallowing by the mouth and the motion of the tongue in the process of chewing.

bone onlay. A length of transplanted bone laid across a break in a bone and held in position by pins, screws, wires, or other means. Used as a permanent splint of a break that eventually becomes incorporated into the bone itself, by the formation of callus.

bone wax. A waxy material used to pack bone in order to stop bone bleeding, especially during operations on the skull.

boss. A knoblike, rounded protuberance at one side of a bone; for example, the mastoid prominence on the skull. May result from disease of the spine.

botulism (*bahch'uh-lihsm*). Germ poisoning resulting from food improperly canned. It is characterized by a sudden severe sickness, weakness, vomiting, diarrhea, and other violent symptoms. It is often fatal.

bougie (*boo'zhih*). A long, slender, cylindrical instrument of waxed silk or rubber or other material used for introduction into various body passages such as the anus, urethra. The instrument is used for exploration of blockages, to increase the diameter of the passage, and as a guide for the passage of other instruments.

bovine. 1. Cattle-like. 2. Derived from, or relating to, a cow or ox as bovine serum, a serum derived from the blood of a cow and used in individuals who are allergic to the more common horse serum.

brachium (*bray'kih-uhm*). The arm, particularly the upper arm; any armlike structure.

bradycardia (*braad-ih-kahr'dih-uh*). Slowness of the heart with the pulse rate less than 60 per minute.

breast. 1. The front of the chest. 2. One of the mammary glands. —*caked b.* Inflammation of the breast following childbirth. —*chicken or pigeon b.* A chest with a prominent breastbone due to rickets or an obstruction of breathing in infancy. —*funnel b.* A chest with a depressed breastbone forming a deep groove. Also due to rickets.

bromhidrosis (*brohm-hih-droh'sihss*). Perspiration with a disagreeable odor.

bromide. Any salt containing bromine. Used as a sedative in nervous conditions; as a pain killer in combination with other drugs; to check convulsions, as in epilepsy. A common bromide is sodium bromide or "triple bromide."

bromine poisoning. Poisoning caused by overuse of bromides. Symptoms are headache, fetid breath, sleepiness, cold extremities, loss of strength and sexual power, shrinkage of the testes and breasts, and an eruption which resembles acne.

bromoderma. A skin eruption due to use of bromides.

bromomania. A psychosis due to prolonged use of bromides.

bronchiectasis (*brahn-kih-ehk'tuh-sihss*). A condition in which the bronchial tubes are ballooned out in certain spots and contain pus and mucus. This condition may exist in one part of a single lung or in many parts of both lungs. It is a debilitating condition with symptoms of breathlessness, cough, and expectoration of large amounts of foul-smelling phlegm containing pus. It is usually due to infection and surgery is often required.

bronchiole (*brahn'kih-ohl*). The smallest subdivision of the breathing tubes within the lung (one millimeter or less in diameter).

bronchiolitis (*brahn-kih-oh-ligh'tihss*). Inflammation of the bronchioles. Also called *capillary bronchitis*.

bronchitis. Inflammation of the lining membrane of the bronchial tubes. There are many types classified according to their cause and symptoms.

bronchogenic (*brahn-kuh-jehn'ihk*). Arising in a bronchus, as bronchogenic cancer (cancer arising in a bronchial tube).

bronchogram. The X-ray of the bronchial tubes made after the inhalation or instillation into the bronchi of a substance which is opaque to X-ray. Usually an iodine-containing oil is introduced into the bronchial tubes by instillation through the nose or throat. The X-ray is taken immediately after such introduction. Since the iodized oil will not permit X-rays to pass through, it outlines the bronchial passages on the film.

bronchography (*brahn-kahg'ruh-fih*). The process by which a bronchogram is made.

bronchopneumonia (*brahn-kuh-noo-moh'nih-uh*). An inflammation of the lung that spreads from infected bronchial tubes. This disease may assume a patchy character throughout the lung, since the bronchial tubes are present everywhere in the lung. In contradistinction to *lobar pneumonia*, where the inflammation is limited to the lobes of the lung. Common in the very young or the very old and caused by a great variety of germs.

bronchoscope. A long tubelike instrument, with a system of mirrors within, introduced into the bronchial tubes for the examination of their interiors.

bronchospasm (*brahn'kuh-spasm*). Narrowing of the bronchial diameter due to violent contraction of the bronchial muscles.

bronchostenosis. Permanent narrowing of the passageways within one or more bronchial tubes.

bronchus. A tubelike branch of the windpipe which divides and subdivides into narrower and narrower tubes, making up the air passages within the lungs.

bronze diabetes. A disease which is characterized by the discoloration of the skin because of deposits of a certain blood pigment. Primarily a disturbance of the liver. The presence of sugar in the urine has given it its name. Also called *hemochromatosis*.

brown mixture. A liquid medicine containing opium and licorice, used to relieve cough.

Brucella. A type of bacillus that causes *undulant fever* in man and contagious abortion in cattle. There are three species of brucella: *b. abortus,* found in the cow; *b. melitensis,* found in the goat; *b. suis,* found in the pig.

brucellergin (*broo-sehl'luhr-jihn*). An extract made from the brucella organism used as a skin test for the diagnosis of undulant fever.

brucellosis. A disease with recurrent attacks of fever caused by infection with the brucella germ. The disease may be acute and of short duration or chronic and of long duration. The general symptoms are weakness, weight loss, thinning of the blood. Any part of the body may be involved. The disease spreads from animal to animal and from animal to man, not uncommonly through the milk or flesh of the animal; it is rarely spread from man to man. Cattle, hogs, goats are the chief sources of infection. Also called *undulant fever, Malta fever, Mediterranean fever*.

bruise. *See* CONTUSION.

bruit (*broo-ee'*). A term used for a particular abnormal sound heard when listening through the stethoscope to the heart or arteries.

bubo (*byou'boh*). An inflammation and swelling of one or more of the glands in the groin or the armpit that usually results in pus formations. Occurs very frequently after one of the venereal diseases.

bulimia. An unusually great and insatiable appetite. Seen often in certain psychoses, diabetes, and brain injuries.

bulla. A large blister.

bunion. A swelling of the lower joint of the large toe associated with a thickening of the skin and an outward turning of the toe.

bunionectomy. The surgical removal of a bunion.

burn. The reaction of tissue to the application of undue heat, caustics, or electricity. Classified as first-degree, where the skin is simply reddened; second-degree, where blisters form; third-degree, where the skin is charred.

bursa. A small fluid-containing balloon of tissue interposed between parts that move upon one another, as *Achilles b.*, a bursa lying between the heel tendon and the heel bone; *prepatellar b.*, a bursa situated over the kneecap.

bursectomy. The surgical removal of a bursa.

bursitis. Inflammation of a bursa accompanied by pain, particularly on movement of the parts involved. A common example of bursitis is the prepatellar bursitis, an inflammation of the bursa in front of the kneecap ordinarily known as "housemaid's knee."

buttock. One of the two fleshy parts of the body just behind the hip joint formed by the masses of the gluteal muscles.

byssinosis (*bihss-ih-noh'sihss*). An irritation of the air passages in the lung due to inhalation of cotton dust.

C

cachexia (*kuh-kehk'sih-uh*). Weakness and extreme weight loss caused by a number of serious diseases, including tuberculosis and cancer.

cachinnation (*kaak-ihn-nay'shuhn*). Immoderate laughter typical of hysteria.

calamine. A pink powder, insoluble in water, made of zinc oxide with a small amount of iron oxide and used as a local application in the treatment of skin diseases, and also to give a flesh color to ointments, washes, and powders.

calcaneus (*kaal-kay'nih-uhss*). The heel bone.

calcareous (*kaal-kaar'ih-uhss*). 1. Related to, or of the nature of, limestone. 2. Having a chalky appearance or consistency. 3. Containing calcium.

calcicosis (*kaal-suh-koh'sihss*). A form of inflammation of the lungs caused by inhalation of marble dust. Common among sculptors, stonecutters, marble quarry workers.

calcification. The deposit of calcium within the tissues of the body. Calcification is a normal process in the formation of bone, or may be abnormal in the healing of tuberculous areas of the lung where calcium is deposited.

calcinosis (*kaal-suh-noh'sihss*). The deposit of calcium in the skin and its underlying tissues resulting from a disorder of the parathyroid glands. May occur as *circumscribed*, limited to the upper extremities (particularly the hands) and seen in a condition called *scleroderma*; or may appear as *diffuse*, where the deposition is widespread with a tendency to ulcerate and involve muscles, tendons, nerves. Seen especially in children. The condition commonly meant when a patient is said to be "turning into stone."

calculus. A small stone composed of mineral substances found in ducts, passages, hollow organs. Examples are kidney stone, gall stone.

calf. The fleshy part of the back of the leg. *See* GASTROCNEMIUS, SOLEUS, and PLANTARIS MUSCLES.

callus. 1. An area of hardened and thickened skin. A reaction to pressure and friction, usually seen in the palm or on the sole, and often accompanied by pain. One of the most common foot ailments caused by badly fitted shoes. 2. Around a break of bone, a *callus* is laid down by the body as the initial stage in uniting the ends of the break.

calomel. Mercurous chloride. A tasteless, white powder formerly used as a purgative, and in the treatment of syphilis.

calorie, calory. A unit of heat. The amount of heat required to raise the temperature of one kilogram of water from 0 to 1 degree centigrade. Most commonly, a unit of measure of the amount of energy derived from food, as one slice of bread yields 100 calories.

calvities (*kaal-vihsh'ih-eez*). Baldness, loss of hair. *See* ALOPECIA.

cancer. Any tumor which by its own structure or properties threatens life.

cancroid. 1. Like cancer. 2. A tumor composed of a special kind of cell known as an *epithelial cell*. 3. A kind of skin cancer, ordinarily not very dangerous.

canker. A small area of ulceration, especially of the mouth and lips, commonly called a canker sore. Usually associated with various infections or stomach upsets.

cantharides (*kaan-thaar'uh-deez*). A drug composed of dried and powdered Spanish Fly (*Cantharis vesicatoria*), an insect whose blistering bite injects *cantharidin*, a poisonous substance. Used locally, redness and blistering result. Internally, cantharides produce irritation, pain, vomiting, severe inflammation of the stomach and intestines, and erection of the penis. Popularly considered an aphrodisiac.

canthus. The angle of the eye, both the inner near the nose, and the outer near the temple.

capillary. The smallest blood vessel that exists in a vast network throughout the body; the connecting channel between the systems of arteries and veins.

capsule. 1. The tissue covering a part, as the liver capsule, the kidney capsule, the joint capsule. 2. An envelope enclosing certain microscopic organisms, as the tuberculosis germ, the germ of sleeping sickness, and others. 3. A soluble shell usually made of gelatin for administering medicines.

caput. The head; also the principal part of the beginning of an organ.

carbohydrate. One of the major classes of food; that class of compounds that includes sugars, dextrines, starches, and cellulose (potatoes, cane sugar, chocolate, bread). Chief and constant constituents are carbon, hydrogen, and oxygen. Carbohydrate foods are used by the body essentially as sources of immediate energy and, in excess, are converted rapidly into stores of fat.

carbuncle. A painful, deep-seated, pus-producing inflammation of the tissues immediately under the skin. A carbuncle is much larger than a boil and has a flat surface, and unlike a boil it discharges pus from many points. Usually a carbuncle is accompanied by fever, weakness, and general sickness. When not successfully treated, the entire area is destroyed and falls away, healing in a scarred crater. Frequently seen on the neck. At times associated with diabetes.

carcinoma (*kahr-sih-noh'muh*). A tumor, or mass of cells that has its origin in the skin or the lining tissue of various organs. These cells are known as *epithelial cells*, with little or no intercellular substance, and are threatening to life. There are various forms of carcinoma, each of which has a different significance in its ability to spread through the body, yield to treatment, and endanger the life of the patient.

cardiac. 1. *a.* Relating to the heart. 2. *n.* A person with a heart disease. 3. *n.* A tonic that acts upon the heart. *See also* CARDIOSPASM.

cardiac failure. Heart failure. The set of symptoms that comes on through failure of the heart as a pumping organ. There are various types of failure depending upon which side of the heart is mostly involved. When the left side of the heart fails, unsatisfactory and difficult breathing is the most prominent symptom. When the right side of the heart fails, all the organs of the body become engorged with blood from the veins, the legs and other parts of the body swell, and fluid accumulates in the abdominal cavity and in the chest. Failure may be due to many conditions: infections such as syphilis and rheumatic fever, hardening of the arteries, high blood pressure.

cardiology. That branch of medicine devoted to the study, diagnosis, and treatment of the heart and its diseases.

cardiophobia. Morbid fear of heart disease.

cardiospasm. A contraction of the muscles controlling the inlet to the stomach. Cardiospasm is often associated with spasm of the upper third of the stomach, and widening and enlargement of the gullet. It is accompanied by severe pain in the upper abdomen or chest and may or may not produce nausea and vomiting.

carotid. The principal large artery on each side of the neck.

carpal. Relating to the wrist.

carpus. The wrist, made up of eight small bones.

cartilage. Gristle.

caseation (*kay-sih-ay′shuhn*). The conversion of tissue into a soft cheese-like substance by certain diseases, as tuberculosis.

casein (*kay'seen*). A protein obtained from milk by the action of acid or an enzyme known as *rennin*. Cheeses contain a high percentage of casein.

castration complex. A fear of castration or injury to the sex organs; symbolizing also fear of injury to the person or his possessions, or separation from any desired person, object, or need. This fear, although influencing the person's actions, attitudes, and feelings, is unknown to the person because it lies below the level of awareness. *See* COMPLEX.

catabolism. The breaking down of complex compounds, such as food, into simpler ones, the destruction of tissue that occurs in day-to-day living, certain diseases, and aging. This process is usually accompanied by the liberation of energy, and is the opposite of *anabolism*. Together catabolism and anabolism constitute *metabolism*.

catalepsy. A morbid, trancelike state in which voluntary motion is lost and the muscles assume a peculiar type of rigidity. Because of this rigidity the patient will retain for an indefinite period of time any position in which he is placed. Catalepsy is seen particularly in hysteria, certain types of insanity (including schizophrenia), and in certain stages of hypnosis.

catalyst. A substance that increases the speed of a chemical reaction without itself being changed during the reaction, as inorganic: heated platinum, in the presence of which hydrogen and oxygen unite to form water, the platinum remaining unchanged; organic: *lipase*, an enzyme of the pancreas, stomach, and intestines that breaks down fats to simpler elements, itself remaining unchanged.

cataplexy. 1. A sudden loss of the normal tension of muscles, the general limpness of an unconscious person. Provoked by an undue emotional experience and often associated with periods of sleep. 2. The prostration that occurs at times by the sudden onset of a disease. 3. Hypnotic sleep.

cataract. Clouding of the lens of the eye that partially or entirely prevents light from entering the eye. There are many types and degrees of cataract. Diabetes, injury to the eye, and old age are the most common causes.

catarrh. A once popular term to identify inflammation of the lining tissue of various organs, particularly of the nose, throat, and air passages, and characeried by an outpouring of mucus.

catatonia. A phase of schizophrenia in which the patient stands or sits in one position, assumes long-enduring postures, and resists any attempt to make him move or talk. A stupor, that may be marked by outbursts of hallucination and panic.

catharsis. 1. Purging. 2. In psychoanalysis, a mental and emotional purge, as intense crying, talking, laughing about a subject long repressed.

cathartic. A medicine that produces evacuation of the bowel, as Epsom salts.

catheter (*kaath'uh-tuhr*). A hollow tube, narrow or wide, made of metal, glass, rubber, or other materials for the introduction into a cavity through its canal. Its purpose is to discharge the fluid contents of a cavity. The relief of accumulated urine within the bladder is made possible by passing a catheter through the urethra.

cathexis (*kuh-thehk'sihss*). The emotional energy attached to an object. It may be positive (as love, desire) or negative (as hate, anxiety), and is particularly conspicuous in pathological cases. For instance, a piece of clothing, usually not emotionally charged, may acquire a cathexis of libido if it belongs to a beloved one. To a fetishist, a lock of hair has a cathexis. Walking across open space carries an anxiety cathexis for one suffering from agoraphobia.

caul. A part of the sac within which the infant develops in the womb and which covers its head on birth.

causalgia (*kaw-zaal'jih-uh*). The burning pain at times appearing in nerve injuries, particularly the nerves of sensation in the palms and on the soles. Often follows frostbite or trench foot.

caustic. A substance that destroys tissue; very irritant; burning. Examples include caustic soda (sodium hydroxide), caustic potash (potassium hydroxide).

cautery. 1. Destruction of tissue by the use of an agent that causes charring. 2. A device or instrument that causes this destructive change. Examples of cautery are the electric sparking-off of small growths on the skin, the use of a chemical, such as silver nitrate, for the same purpose, and the use of a hot-tipped instrument.

cavernous. Having hollow spaces.

cecostomy (*see-kahs'tuh-mih*). Establishing an artificial opening into the large intestine near the appendix. This opening connects with other areas of the intestine and is made as a shunt around diseased loops of the intestine.

cecum (*see'kuhm*). The first part of the large intestine. From its lowermost and blind end the appendix hangs.

centrifuge. 1. *n*. An apparatus for separating substances of different densities by rapid spinning. 2. *v*. To separate substances by spinning.

cephalalgia (*seh-fuh-laal'jih-uh*). Headache.

cephalic (*seh-faal'ihk*). Relating to the head.

cerebellum (*seh-reh-behl'luhm*). The lower back part of the brain that controls body balance and muscular co-ordination.

cerebration. Mental activity.

cerebrum (*sehr'ee-bruhm*). The main part of the brain that occupies the entire upper part of the skull and is divided into a right and left hemisphere.

cerumen (*seh-roo'muhn*). Earwax.

cervicectomy (*suhr-vuh-sehk'tuh-mih*). Amputation of the neck of the womb.

cervicitis (*suhr-vuh-sigh'tihss*). Inflammation of the neck of the womb.

cervix. A narrow portion or neck. Most commonly refers to the neck of the womb.

Caesarian section. An incision through the abdominal wall and the womb for delivery of an infant.

chalazion (*kuh-lay'zih-uhn*). A tumor of the eyelid, resulting from accumulated fluid in the small glands (*Meibomian glands*) beneath the lining tissue of the lid.

chancre (*shaan'kuhr*). Usually refers to the first noticeable sign of syphilis that appears as a painless ulcer at the point of contact. Most often the chancre is upon the penis or within the vagina.

chancroid (*shaan'kroyd*). A painful ulceration involving the genitalia usually caused by a specific venereal disease. Commonly called *soft chancre*.

chaulmoogra oil (*shuhl-moo'gruh*). A yellow oil obtained from the seeds of certain trees of Burma and India used in the treatment of leprosy.

cheilitis (*kigh-ligh'tihss*). Inflammation of the lips through a number of causes, such as sunlight, poison oils, allergy.

cheilosis (*kigh-loh'sihss*). A disorder of the lips caused by vitamin deficiency. Early, the angles of the lips are pale; scaling and thickening follow, and then deep cracks appear. Also called *riboflavin deficiency*.

chemosis. Swelling of the lining membrane of the lids and eyes.

chemotherapy (*kehm-oh-thehr'uh-pih*). The treatment or prevention of diseases by chemicals that act to destroy or inactivate the condition, without causing any poisonous effect in the patient. Sulfa drugs are chemotherapeutic.

chicken pox. A contagious disease of childhood characterized by an eruption of small, itchy blisters occurring in crops on various parts of the body. Also called *varicella*.

chigger. A developing mite of a certain insect (*trombicula*). The bite of the chigger causes severe inflammation.

chilblain. Swelling and congestion of the skin with severe itching or burning. Blisters may form and develop into ulceration. Caused by exposure to cold. Other names are *erythema pernio* or *pernio*.

chirology (*kigh-rahl'uh-jih*). Method of communicating with deaf mutes by means of the hands.

chloasma (*kloh-aaz'muh*). Patches of pigment in the skin of various sizes and shapes, yellow, brown, or black in color. Often associated with certain glandular derangements. Other names are *melanoderma* and *melasma*. —*c. hepaticum*. Liver spots. Popularly used to denote any pigmentation of the face and chest. —*c. phthisicorum*. Found in tuberculous patients as brown patches of the forehead or upper parts of the cheeks. —*c. uterinum*. Patches on the forehead, temples, cheeks, nipples, and abdomen. These patches may be made more intense by pregnancy, menstruation, disorders of the ovary, and various derangements of the womb.

chloromycetin (*klaw-ruh-migh-see'tuhn*). One of the new antibiotics obtained from a soil fungus known as *streptomyces*.

chlorosis. A form of anemia most common in young women, characteried by a greenish tinge to the skin.

cholagogue (*koh'luh-gahg*). Any agent that stimulates the flow of bile; for example, eating of fats.

cholangitis (*koh-laan-jigh'tihss*). Inflammation of the biliary ducts, tiny canals within the liver through which the bile flows.

cholecystectomy (*koh-luh-sihss-tehk'tuh-mih*). Surgical removal of the gall bladder.

cholecystitis (*koh-luh-sihss-tigh'tihss*). Inflammation of the gall bladder.

cholecystogram (*koh-luh-sihss'toh-gram*). X-ray picture of the gall bladder.

cholecystography (*koh-luh-sihss-tahg'ruh-fih*). X-ray of the gall bladder after the patient has swallowed, or been injected with, a material opaque to X-ray that finds its way into the gall bladder. By this means the gall bladder is outlined on the X-ray picture.

cholelith. A stone in the bile duct or gall bladder.

cholemia. The presence of bile in the blood.

cholera. An acute, serious, infectious disease characterized by severe diarrhea, with watery stools, vomiting, muscular cramps, lack of urination, and collapse. A terrible scourge, particularly of the Far East, where it appears in epidemic form. Fatalities are numerous. It is spread through food or water and is caused by a germ known as *vibrio comma* (shaped like a comma).

cholesterol (*koh-lehss'tuh-rahl*). A substance that is a constituent of all animal fats and oils, of bile, gallstones, egg yolk, nervous system tissue, and blood. Cholesterol is related in some unknown fashion to hardening of the arteries, high blood pressure, stone formation, and other diseases. It is important in the over-all metabolism of the body and can be stimulated to produce a form of vitamin D.

choline (*koh'leen*). An important substance with a crystalline base, widely distributed in plants and animals, containing nitrogen. It is thought to be a member of the vitamin B complex. An important derivative of choline is *acetylcholine*, which plays a primary role in the transmission of nervous impulses.

cholinesterase (*koh-lih-nehss'tuh-rayss*). An enzyme that is found in the blood and other parts of the body, which neutralizes *acetylcholine*. Because of this action it, too, is important in the transmission of nervous impulses.

choluria (*koh-loo'rih-uh*). The presence of bile in the urine.

chondral (*kahn'druhl*). Relating to cartilage or gristle.

chondroma. A tumor that resembles cartilage. May arise from bone, cartilage, or other tissues; usually is not serious but tends to recur after removal.

chordee (*kawr-dee'*). A painful, curved erection of the penis, with concavity downward. Usually due to gonorrhea.

chorea (*kaw-ree'uh*). A nervous disorder that may be a disease itself or may result from specific diseases. It is characterized by irregular, uncontrollable movements of the muscles of the legs, arms, and face. Other names are *Sydenham's chorea, St. Vitus dance, dancing chorea, choromania.*

choriomeningitis (*kaw-rih-oh-meh-nihn-jigh'tihss*). An inflammation of the coverings of the brain, particularly the middle and internal layers.

chorion (*kawr'ih-ahn*). The outermost of the several layers of tissue that make up the sac within the womb in which the infant develops.

choroid. A layer of the eyeball that is continuous with the colored part of the eye in front, and extends around the eyeball to its hindmost portion. Consisting of many blood vessels, it is the middle layer of the eyeball, lying between the tough, fibrous outer layer seen in front of the eye as the eye-white, the *sclera*, and the inner hindlayer of nervous tissues, known as the *retina*.

choroiditis (*kohr-oy-digh'tihss*). Inflammation of the choroid, the middle layer of the eyeball. Choroiditis takes on varied forms, according to its cause, to the area of choroid involved, and to the presence or absence of pus.

chromatelopsia (*kroh-muh-teh-lahp'sih-uh*). Color blindness.

chromatosis. 1. Pigmentation. 2. A disease process in which coloring matter is deposited in areas where it usually does not exist, or in unusual amounts in areas where it ordinarily does occur.

chronic. Long continued; of long duration.

chyle (*kighl*). A milk-white emulsion of fat globules, formed in the small intestine during digestion, finding its way into the lymph. A stage in the digestion of fat.

chyme (*kighm*). The thick liquid contents of the stomach that have undergone digestion and have not yet been passed into the small intestine.

cicatrix (*sihk'uh-trihks*). A scar. The scar tissue that replaces the tissue lost through injury or disease. When new, the scar tissue is reddish or purple; when old, it is white and glistening.

cinchona (*sihn-koh'nuh*). The bark of a tree native to South America from which quinine is made.

circulation time. The rate of blood flow. This time is computed by injecting a small quantity of material that has a specific taste or odor into an arm vein and noting the time it takes between injection and the patient's stated awareness of the taste or odor.

cirrhosis (*sih-roh'sihss*). A long-standing inflammation of the liver that may lead to its enlargement or shrinkage and perhaps to death. There are many varieties of cirrhosis caused by a number of conditions, among them heart disease, alcoholic poisoning, obstruction of bile ducts, and various infections such as syphilis and others.

cirsectomy (*suhr-sehk'tuh-mih*). Surgical removal of a part of a varicose vein.

cisvestitism (*sihss-vehss'tih-tihsm*). Dressing in clothes of one's own sex, but inappropriate to one's age, or station in life; for example, an adult dressing as a child.

claudication. Lameness. —*intermittent c.* Weakness and cramp-like pain in the legs, particularly the calves. At times associated with excessive smoking.

clavicle. The collar bone, the prominent bone on the upper part of each side of the chest just below the neck that attaches to the breastbone.

clavus. A corn.

climacteric. Change of life. A period in which the system undergoes marked changes. In women, characterized by a gradual stoppage of menstruation, at times emotional disturbances, and the acquisition of minor secondary sex characteristics of the male, such as a hairy growth in the beard area, a deepening of the voice, a shrinkage of the breast, and others.

climatotherapy. The treatment of disease by means of a change to a suitable climate.

clinical. Relating to bedside treatment. Pertaining to the signs, symptoms, and the course of a disease, as observed by the physician, and opposed to changes noted in the laboratory and under a microscope.

clitoris (*kliht'uh-rihss*). An erective part of the female genital situated in the upper fold formed by the lips of the vagina; resembling the penis in the male; the site of many nerves of sensation.

clitorism. 1. Enlargement of the clitoris. 2. A condition of painful and persistent erection of the clitoris, similar to the painful, persistent erection of the penis in the male.

clonus. Spasm of muscles, characterized by involuntary alternate contractions and relaxation. Clonus can be induced, for example, in the wrist or the ankle by rapid back and forth movement of these joints by the examiner.

clotting time. The time required for clotting of a small amount of blood obtained by puncturing the skin. An important test to determine certain characteristics of the blood. Normal clotting time is about ten minutes.

clubfoot. *See* TALIPES VARUS.

coagulant. 1. Causing the formation of a clot. 2. Any agent that causes the formation of a clot.

coagulate. 1. To curdle; clot. 2. To change from a liquid to a compact, jelly-like mass resembling the formation of gelatine in a cooling atmosphere.

coalescence. The union of two or more things previously separate, as two small areas of skin rash, growing larger and becoming one area.

coarctation (*koh-ahrk-tay'shuhn*). The narrowing of a tube at one point, giving it the appearance of an hourglass. This narrowing occurs in blood vessels, particularly the main artery that comes from the heart, the aorta.

coccidioidomycosis (*kahk-sih-dih-oy-doh-migh-koh'sihss*). A disease caused by the inhalation of spores of a fungus known as *Coccidioides immitis*. The symptoms are many and varied and have often been confused with tuberculosis. The disease involves primarily the lungs and the skin, although many other organs and systems are known to be involved. Commonly called *San Joaquin Valley fever*. Seen in great numbers among desert-trained troops in World War II.

coccygectomy (*kahk-sih-jehk'tuh-mih*). Surgical removal of the coccyx, the tail bone, the very lowest end of the spine.

coccygodynia (*kahk-sih-goh-dihn'ih-uh*). Pain in the region of the coccyx, tail bone.

coccyx (*kahk'sihks*). The last bone of the spinal column formed by the union of four rudimentary vertebrae. The tail bone.

cochlea (*kahk'lih-uh*). A cavity in the internal ear that resembles a snail shell. This cavity contains the important organs of hearing, which transform the vibrations received via the outer and middle ear into nervous impulses that are transmitted to the brain for translation into sound.

coitus (*koh'ih-tuhss*). The act of sexual intercourse; copulation. —*c. interruptus*. Sexual intercourse in which the penis is withdrawn and the semen discharged outside the vagina.

colectomy. The surgical removal of a part of the large intestine.

colic. 1. Relating to the colon or large intestine. 2. Pain in the abdomen coming in attacks caused by spasm of the intestinal muscles. Colic is a symptom of a host of conditions, such as appendicitis, obstruction of the gall bladder opening by a stone, lead poisoning, overeating, or emotional disturbance.

colitis. Inflammation of the large intestine. Colitis may be of a number of types each due to infection by specific organisms. Characterized according to specific symptoms, as *mucus c.*, where the stool contains threads or masses of tissue and mucus.

collyrium. A local medicated application to the eye, usually a wash or a lotion.

colon. That part of the large intestine which begins at the cecum and ends at the rectum; the length of intestine between the small intestine and the rectum.

colostomy (*koh-lahs'tuh-mih*). A permanent opening established through the abdominal wall into the large intestine, as an artificial anus. Made in those cases where the rectum and anus are diseased or eradicated because of disease.

colostrum. The initial milk from the mother's breast after childbirth. The composition of colostrum is different from the ordinary breast milk. Its purpose is laxative in order to assist the expulsion of the infant's intestinal content.

colpalgia (*kahl-paal'jih-uh*). Vaginal pain, or neuralgia.

colpaltitis. Inflammation of the vagina.

colpectomy. Surgical excision of the vagina.

colpocele (*kahl'poh-seel*). A tumor or a rupture into the vagina.

colpoplasty. A plastic operation of the vagina.

colpotomy. An incision of the vagina.

coma. A state of unconsciousness from which the patient cannot be aroused. Follows brain tumor, injury, apoplexy; poisoning, as with narcotics, alcohol, or poisons developed in the body by disease; disturbance of the chemical balance in the body as in uncontrolled diabetes.

comatose. State of being in a coma.

comedo (*kahm'uh-doh*). A blackhead. A collection of oil and dead cells in the oil glands of the skin, the duct of which is covered with a dark crust, usually found on the face, chest, and back. Most common in adolescence.

comminute (*kahm'mih-nyout*). A bone broken so that it is shattered in several pieces.

commitment. Act of consigning a patient to an institution.

common cold. An acute infection of the nose, throat, voice box, and at times the breathing tubes, because of a virus. After the virus invades these areas, "secondary invaders" (as the streptococcus, staphylococcus, pneumococcus, influenza bacillus) make their appearance. The common cold is usually mild, of short duration, highly contagious. Characterized by sudden onset of chilliness, sneezing, tears, nasal discharge, cough, and fever. Also called *coryza, upper respiratory infection, rhinitis.*

complex. A group of ideas with their charges of emotional energy, which, because they are opposed to the energy charges of another group of ideas with resulting conflict,

have been pushed below the level of awareness into the unconscious.

compress. A cloth folded, or a pad, or other soft material,
dry or wet, that is applied to a part of the body for the
relief of inflammation or the prevention of hemorrhage.

concha (*kahn'kuh*). A shell-like organ, as the outer ear.

condom. A sheath worn over the penis during intercourse
for preventing conception or infection.

condyloma (*kahn-dih-loh'muh*). A wartlike growth or small
tumor near the anus or genitals.

confabulation. Ready recitals of fictitious occurrences found
in certain mental disorders.

conflict. The battle between opposing forces in the mind, one
of which is often repressed.

congenital. Existing at birth.

congestion. An abnormal collection of blood in a part of an
organ.

conjunctiva (*kahn-juhnk-tigh'vuh*). The tissue lining the
visible part of the eye and the under surfaces of both lids.

conjunctivitis (*kahn-juhnk-tih-vigh'tihss*). Inflammation of
the conjunctiva that may be due to many causes such as infection, allergy, irritation. Named according to cause, severity, appearance, seasonal occurrence. Pinkeye is an example.

contracture. 1. A shortening of tissue, as of a muscle or scar
tissue, that produces deformity or distortion. Examples are
scars on face, or drawing down of the eye, the lips to one
side, the nose out of line. 2. Retarded relaxation of muscle.

contre-coup (*kawn-truh-koo'*). The injury of a part opposite to the one that is struck due to transmission of the shock.
Example: A break in the bone of the skull on the side opposite to that which received the injury.

contusion. A bruise or an injury in which the skin is not
broken.

convulsant. Medicine that causes convulsions, as insulin used
for shock in mental patients.

convulsion. An uncontrollable contraction of muscles over large areas of the body. This contraction may be periodic, alternating with relaxation of the muscles, or there may be no relaxation of muscles. There are many varieties of convulsions, such as in epilepsy, birth injury, childbirth fever, poisons of various sorts. Convulsion may occur with or without the loss of consciousness.

corn. *See* CLAVUS.

cornea (*kawr'nih-uh*). The transparent front covering of the eyeball, part of the white of the eye, through which is seen *the pupil* and its surrounding colored portion, *the iris*.

corneum. The outmost layer of skin.

cornification. The process by which skin is converted into such derivatives as hair, nails, feathers; or becomes hornlike as in calluses. When a new fingernail is grown, cornification occurs.

coronary. A word used to indicate blood vessels or nerves or other attachments to a part that entirely encircle it. Loosely used to mean *c. thrombosis* or a clot in an important blood vessel of the heart that may kill or incapacitate the patient. C. thrombosis is most frequent in males of middle age; a severe pressure pain, vise-like in character in the chest, shoots into the shoulder and down the left arm and fingers.

corpuscle. An archaic term for a cell, especially a blood cell; any small rounded body.

cortex. The outer layer of the brain, "the grey matter"; also the outer portion of an organ immediately below its capsule.

cortisone. A hormone derived from the outer portion of the adrenal gland, found to be useful in treating many conditions, especially some types of arthritis. Also called *compound E*.

coruscation. The sensation of flashes of light before the eyes. Epileptics and those with migraine often experience this symptom. The common "seeing stars" when injured.

coryza (*kuh-righ'zuh*). Nasal catarrh. *See also* COMMON COLD.

costalgia. Pain in the ribs.

costectomy. Surgical removal of part of, or an entire rib.

counter irritant. Any agent that causes an inflammation of the skin for the relief of a deep-seated inflammation. For example, the mustard plaster applied to the chest for relief of congestion of the lungs.

coxa. The hip or the hip joint.

coxalgia (*kahk-saal'jih-uh*). Pain in the hip or disease of the hip joint.

cramp. 1. A painful spasm of a muscle, as occurs in the legs of runners. 2. Spasmodic pain, as in the gut during a stomach upset. 3. Paralysis of certain muscles that comes and goes. 4. Painful menstruation.

cranium. The part of the skull that contains the brain and its coverings.

crapulent, crapulous. Characterized by excessive eating and drinking.

cravat. A triangular-shaped bandage used as a temporary wound dressing or for the support of a broken bone.

creatine (*kree'uh-tihn*). An important organic compound found in many animal tissues, particularly in muscle. Strategic in the process of muscular contraction.

creatinine (*krih-aat'ih-nihn*). A substance normally found in the blood and urine and excreted in the urine at a constant rate as a by-product of creatine usage in the muscular system of the body.

cremaster (*krih-maass'tuhr*). The muscle that draws up the testis.

crenation. Used particularly to describe red blood cells when exposed to the air or strong salt solution. The cells shrink and take on a notched or cogwheel appearance.

crepitation. 1. The grating sound of broken bones when the ends rub against each other. 2. The crackling of joints. 3. The noise that is made when air is captured under the skin or within tissues; the air captured in the skin by gas gangrene infections would be an example. 4. The sound heard through the stethoscope at the end of an inhalation during certain lung conditions. Pieces of crumpled tissue paper rubbed together give a similar sound.

cretinism. A condition due to severe deficiency of the thyroid gland. Appears at or before birth or in early infancy. Cretinism is characterized by a large protruding tongue, dry thick skin, protruding abdomen, the mentality of an idiot, and the physical size of a dwarf. It is common in certain areas of the world where there is a lack of iodine in the food or water supply. Varying degrees of this condition at one time were very common around the Great Lakes regions in the United States.

cross-eye. *See* STRABISMUS.

croup. A condition of the voice box in children that results in a harsh, crowing cough and difficulty in breathing. There are many types of croup due to a number of conditions, such as injury to the voice box, diphtheria, and others.

cryptogenic (*krihp-tuh-jehn'ihk*). Of unknown or obscure cause.

cryptorchidectomy (*krihp-tawr-kih-dehk'tuh-mih*). The surgical removal of a testis that has failed to descend into the scrotum.

cryptorchidopexy (*krihp-tawr-kih-duh-pehk'sih*). Anchoring within the scrotum by surgical sewing of a testis that has not normally descended into the sac.

cryptorchism (*krihp-tawr'kihzm*). A defect in development in which the testes fail to descend from the abdomen into the scrotum. The normal process during development within the mother's womb is for the testes to form in the abdominal cavity and gradually descend through the inguinal canal, in the region of the groin, into their natural position within the scrotal sac.

curare (*kyou-rah'rih*). A drug that paralyzes the muscles by preventing nervous impulses from reaching them. In excess dosage this drug may cause death by suffocation because of paralysis of the muscles required in breathing. Curare is used medically to control convulsions and muscular spasms, especially in the treatment of certain nervous disorders. It is also used to relax the muscles when a general anaesthetic is given. In South America particularly, it is used as an arrow poison by the aborigines.

curarization (*kyou-ruh-rih-zay'shuhn*). Placing a subject under the full influence of curare. The power of motion and speech disappears but sensitivity to pain remains.

curettage (*kyou-reh-tahj'*). Scraping the interior of a cavity by finger or with a curette.

curette (*kyou-reht'*). A spoon- or scoop-shaped metal instrument used for scraping away dead tissue. This instrument is commonly used in performing an abortion.

cutaneous (*kyou-tay'nih-uhss*). Relating to the skin.

cuticle. A horny, thickened layer formed by, and covering the top cells of, the skin.

cutis. The skin.

cyanosis (*sigh-uh-noh'sihss*). A bluish tinge of the skin and lining tissues resulting from the absence of a sufficient quantity of usable oxygen in the blood. An example is the blue face in suffocation associated with strangling, heart failure, severe pneumonia.

cyclothymia (*sigh-kluh-thigh'mih-uh*). A condition characterized by alternating states of elation and depression. The most severe form is known as manic-depressive psychosis.

cyesis (*sigh-ee'sihss*). Pregnancy.

cyst. Actually means a bladder; that is, a sac or pouch with a distinct wall containing fluid or other material. A cyst may be normal, as the urinary bladder or the gall bladder, or it may be abnormal, as in tumor growths containing large amounts of liquid. Cysts are named according to location, contents, and cause.

cystectomy (*sihs-tehk'tuh-mih*). 1. The surgical removal of the duct that leads from the gall bladder to the intestine. 2. Removal of the gall bladder or part of the urinary bladder. 3. Removal of a cyst.

cystography. X-ray of the urinary bladder after it has been

injected with a substance that is opaque to X-ray and outlines the bladder on the X-ray film.

cystoscope. A tubular, hollow instrument bearing a lighting
system and lenses with room for the passage of instruments
used for operation. Employed in diagnosis and treatment of
bladder, kidney, and ureter (the tube that leads from the
kidney to the bladder) conditions.

cytopathology. The branch of medicine that deals with
changes within cells. For example, the examination of cell
specimens from the vagina to determine the presence of
cancer.

D

dacryocystitis (*daak-rih-oh-sihss-tigh′tihss*). Inflammation of
the tear sac in the inner angle of the eye.

dacryorrhea (*daak-rih-aw-ree′uh*). An excessive flow of
tears.

dacryosolenitis (*daak-rih-oh-sohl-eh-nigh′tihss*). Inflammation of the tear duct that leads from the corner of the eye
into the nose.

dacryostenosis (*daak-rih-oh-steh-noh′sihss*). Narrowing of
a tear duct (resulting in interference with the normal flow
of tears).

dactylitis (*daak-tih-ligh′tihss*). Inflammation of a finger or
toe.

dactylus (*daak′tih-luhss*). A finger or toe.

dandruff. Scales from the scalp.

death rattle. A gurgling sound caused by the passage of air
through accumulated fluid in the windpipe; heard in dying
persons.

decalcification. A decrease in the normal mineral salts content of bone. Occurs in certain conditions; such as disease of the parathyroid glands, old age.

decerebration. Removal of the brain. Ordinarily refers to removal of the brain of animals in certain laboratory experiments.

decidua (*dih-sihd'joo-uh*). That part of the lining membrane of the interior of the womb that changes its character in preparation for, and during, pregnancy. The decidua is cast off after childbirth and during menstruation as clots and pieces of tissue.

decompensation. The failure of an organ to adjust itself to changing conditions in order to carry on normal function, as failure of the heart or kidneys in disease and old age.

decompression. The removal of pressure, especially the pressure within the skull cavity. Pressure in the skull cavity becomes high during the course of a tumor growth or bleeding. Decompression is performed by boring a small hole in the skull, commonly in the region of the temple.

decubitus (*dih-kyou'bih-tuhs*). The lying down or horizontal posture. Ulcers or bedsores developing upon patients who are in decubitus (confined to bed for a long time) are called *d. ulcers.*

defloration. The loss of those characteristics that indicate virginity in women. Rupture of the hymen at the first intercourse. The surgical removal of the hymen is not considered defloration.

deglutition. The act of swallowing.

dehydration. The removal of water, as from the body or a tissue. Dehydration may occur through excessive perspiration, diarrhea, or vomiting.

delirium. A condition occurring in various diseases, or following the use of drugs or alcohol. Delirium is characterized by: confusion; excitement; clouded perception; and often hallucinations, illusions, and delusions. The most commonly known type. *d. tremens*, is associated with alcoholic poisoning.

deltoid. 1. The thick, triangular large muscle that covers the shoulder joint and that is attached to the upper third of the armbone. 2. The area covered by the deltoid muscle: the upper, outer part of the arm. 3. Triangular, as the Greek letter Delta.

delusion. A belief maintained despite absolute evidence to the contrary. A frequently seen type is the *delusion of grandeur*, in which the erroneous belief maintained has to do with power, genius, or wealth.

dementia. Deterioration of intelligence, such as the reasoning power, memory, and will. Dementia is characterized by apathy; confusion; unawareness of time, place, distance; and, at times, stupor. Dementia is caused by a number of conditions, such as prolonged use of alcohol, bleeding into the brain, brain fever, and schizophrenia, a type of insanity.

demineralization. The loss of mineral salts from the body, as from the bone. *See decalcification.*

demorphinization. Treatment of morphine addiction by gradual reduction of the amount of drug used.

demulcent. 1. Reducing the irritation, or soothing surfaces, particularly of the lining tissue of various organs. 2. A soothing substance, especially a slippery, gluey liquid.

dengue (*den'ghih*). An epidemic infectious disease caused by a virus carried by certain mosquitoes. Characterized by attacks of fever; severe pain in the bones and muscles; pain, swelling and reddening of the joints. An eruption of the skin may appear. The convalescence is slow. Dengue is particularly widespread through the tropics and subtropics. It is also called *breakbone fever, dandy fever.*

denigration. The process of becoming black. Occurs in certain diseases, particularly Addison's disease, that is a disease of the outer portion of the adrenal glands.

denture. All of the teeth together considered as a unit. Most commonly refers to artificial teeth, complete or partial sets.

depersonalization. A feeling of being someone else; a loss of the sense of one's own reality or identity.

depilate. To remove the hair.

dermatitis. Any inflammation of the skin.

dermatologist. A skin specialist.

dermatology. That branch of medicine that deals with the structure and function of the skin, and its diseases and their treatment.

dermatome. An instrument for cutting long strips of skin for use in skin grafting.

dermatophytid (*duhr-muh-toh-figh'tihd*). A skin rash caused by an allergy to a fungus.

dermatophytosis (*duhr-muh-toh-figh-toh'sihss*). An eruption of the skin characterized by tiny blisters, cracking, and scaling, on the hands and feet, especially between the toes. Also called *ringworm* or *athlete's foot*.

dermatosis. Any disease of the skin.

dermographia. A condition in which the skin is very sensitive to irritation. Often called the "blackboard skin" because a name written with the fingernail upon the skin becomes evident in welts in a few minutes.

dermoid. Resembling skin. Used loosely when referring to a *dermoid cyst*, a tumor containing some of the skin appendages, such as hair.

desensitization. To cause loss of sensitivity or susceptibility. Often used to mean the injection treatment given in allergy, as in hay fever, which results in a gradual reduction of sensitivity to whatever the patient is allergic. More accurately, desensitization describes the same process in animal experiments where sensitivity is totally lost. The proper word for the injection treatment of allergy in man is *hyposensitization*.

desiccant. *n.* A drying medicine, or application. *adj.* Tending to cause drying.

detergent. *n.* 1. An application used for cleansing wounds.

2. A synthetic material used as a soap substitute. *adj.* Cleansing or purifying.

dextrocardia. The presence of the heart in the right side of the chest, instead of the left or normal position.

dextrophobia. A morbid fear of objects on the right side of the body.

diabetes. A disease characterized by the discharge of a large quantity of urine and by unusual thirst. Usually refers to *diabetes mellitus.* —*d. insipidus.* A disease resulting from a disorder of an area of the brain. D. insipidus may appear at birth or follow disease or injury of the brain. Characterized by the discharge of great quantities of urine that resembles water and intense thirst. This disease is relieved by treatment with injections of pituitary gland extracts. —*d. mellitus.* A disease of unknown cause whose chief characteristic is the failure of the body to use carbohydrates at a normal rate. In this condition there is a deficiency of insulin. D. mellitus is characterized by an excess of sugar in the blood, the presence of sugar in the urine, thirst, loss of weight, and weakness. Complications later in life may be hardening of the arteries, inflammation of the nerves, cataracts of the eyes.

diagnosis. 1. The process by which the nature of a disease is determined. 2. The decision reached.

diagnostician. One skilled in determining the nature of a disease.

diaphragm (*digh'uh-fraam*). 1. A partition made up of muscle and tendon, as the partition that separates the chest cavity from the abdominal cavity, an important muscle of breathing; the partition that separates the front of the eye from the lens, the iris, or the colored portion of the eye. 2. A device, usually made of rubber, inserted into the vagina in order to wall off the neck of the womb and thus prevent conception. *See* PESSARY.

diaphysis (*digh-aaf'ih-sihss*). The shaft of a long bone as the arm bone, the thighbone, the shinbone.

diarrhea. Looseness of the bowels characterized by increased frequency and wateriness of the stools.

diastole (*digh-aass'tuh-lee*). The period of relaxation of the heart during which it fills with blood.

diathermy. An oscillating electric current of high frequency used to produce heat in a particular area beneath the skin in the treatment of certain disorders, as low back pain, neuralgia, and others.

dietotherapy. The use of a diet regimen for treatment purposes.

digitalis (*dih-jih-taal'ihss*). A medicine made of the dry leaf of a plant, the common foxglove. Introduced in 1785 by Dr. Withering of Shropshire, England. It is a powerful heart stimulant and is used particularly where the heart is threatening to fail, or has already failed.

digitalization. The initial administration of digitalis in high enough dosages to obtain a beneficial effect, and thereafter in relatively small daily amounts to maintain this effect.

dilatation. 1. The state of being stretched. 2. Enlargement or increase in diameter, as of a hollow part or organ. An example is dilatation of the colon, the marked stretching of the large intestine that ordinarily appears at birth, called *Hirschsprung's disease.*

dionism (*digh'uh-nihsm*). Homosexuality.

diphtheria. A communicable disease caused by the diphtheria germ. Characterized usually by pain, swelling and obstruction in the throat due to the production of false tissue by the germ, fever, prostration, at times injury to the heart, at times paralysis of muscles, and often death.

diplegia (*digh-plee'jih-uh*). Paralysis of similar parts on two sides of the body, such as paralysis of both legs, paralysis of both arms, paralysis of both eyes.

diplopia (*dih-ploh'pih-uh*). Double vision, that is, a single object being seen as two. May result from disturbances within the eyes or elsewhere in the body, or to various poisonings, such as the excessive use of alcohol.

dipsomania. The recurrent, periodic compulsion to excessive alcoholic drinking. The dipsomaniac is the person who every so often locks himself in his room and consumes a case of liquor over a period of several days. Between these binges he may not drink at all.

disarticulation. The separation of bones at a joint, or the amputation of a part at its joint.

disc, disk. A platelike structure or organ. Discs of cartilage normally exist between the bodies of the vertebrae for their easy movement upon one another. A *slipped disc* is a condition ordinarily in the lower spine where one of the discs has slipped out of place causing severe pain in the low back that shoots down the back of the leg into the heel. It is very incapacitating and may appear on simply bending in a certain position. Often requires surgery.

discrete. Separate; not running together, as widely separated hives or pimples.

disease. A sickness, malady, or ailment. A disturbance in the performance or structure of a part or organ of the body.

disinfectant. Any agent that destroys or stops the action of disease-causing germs.

disinfestation. The extermination of parasites, such as worms and insects.

disorientation. The inability to comprehend time, place, and people; loss of the usual orientation or relationship to one's surroundings, and one's own identity. May occur in various emotional disturbances, fever, brain diseases.

displacement. The process by which the energy inherent in an emotion or idea is transferred to an associated idea; an important unconscious method for the production of various symptoms including phobias. Example: A person has a morbid fear of knives to such an extent that it is impossible for him to go into a house where he knows there is a knife. Such an idea controls the person's life even though he knows it is ridiculous. Psychoanalysis reveals that the fear of the knife may represent a wish for his mother's death, which was so horrendous a thought that it was pushed into the unconscious.

distention. A state of widening or enlargement, as the gaseous distention of the gut in "bloating."

diuresis (*digh-you-ree'sihss*). An increased excretion of urine.

diuretic (*digh-you-reht'ihk*). 1. (*adj.*) Increasing the output of urine. 2. (*n.*) Any agent that induces such output. Diuretics are used in those conditions where the volume of urine is decreased due to disease, as in heart failure.

diverticulum (*digh-vuhr-tihk'yuh-luhm*). A pouch that arises from a hollow organ or structure. A diverticulum may exist from birth due to defects in development, or may arise later as the result of disease. Occurs in the gullet, stomach, intestines, bladder, joints, and many other areas. How serious a diverticulum is depends upon its position; whether or not it interferes with function; and whether or not it becomes inflamed. For example, a diverticulum of the gullet may receive and accumulate swallowed food, give it back, and cause coughing and the expulsion of food. This condition may interfere with eating, result in aspiration into the lungs of the retained food, and cause choking and/or serious pneumonia. Such a diverticulum requires operation.

dizziness. *See* VERTIGO.

dorsal. Referring to the back or hind part of an organ.

dorsalgia (*dawr-saal'jih-uh*). Pain in the back.

dorsum. 1. The back. 2. The back of any part, such as the dorsum of the foot or hand.

douche (*doosh*). 1. A stream of water or air directed into a body cavity or against the body itself. Examples include the needle showers of alternating hot and cold water (Scotch douche), the cleansing of the vagina with liquid medication, nasal douches, throat douches, rectal douches, ear douches.

drain. 1. *n.* Material such as rubber tissue, tubing, and gauze that is placed in a wound and led to the exterior of the body to form a channel for exit of discharge. 2. *v.* To discharge accumulated fluid from a cavity by operation or puncture, as removal of "water on the knee" by withdrawing the water via needle and syringe.

dressing. 1. *v.* Applying various materials, as sterile gauze, to protect and favor the healing of a wound. 2. *n.* The materials so used.

dropsy. The collection of fluid under the skin, within other tissues, or in body cavities, such as the chest and abdomen. May result from starvation, heart disease, kidney disease, and other conditions.

duct. A tube or channel that conducts fluid, especially the secretion of a gland. There are numerous ducts in the body such as the *bile duct*, the *duct of the pancreas, milk ducts, tear ducts*, the *ducts of the salivary glands.*

duipara (*doo-ihp'uh-ruh*). A woman who has given birth to two children.

duodenum (*doo-uh-dee'nuhm*). The first eight to ten inches of the small intestine. The duodenum arises from the lower end of the stomach, and contains the opening of the bile duct and the duct from the pancreas.

dura mater. The tough, outermost covering of the brain and spinal cord.

dust count. The number of particles of dust in the air less than one one-hundred-thousandth of an inch in diameter, per cubic foot of air. The dust count is most frequently made to determine the hazards of various trades in which dust is particularly heavy.

dysacousia (*dihss-uh-koo'zhuh*). A condition in which pain or discomfort is caused by even moderate noise.

dysarthria (*dihss-ahr'thrih-uh*). Stammering; impairment of speech.

dysarthrosis. The dislocation, disease, or deformity of a joint.

dyschizia (*dihss-kigh'zih-uh*). Painful or difficult bowel movement.

dyschondroplasia (*dihss-kahn-druh-play'zih-uh*). A disease of unknown cause in which the normal hardening of gristle into bone is long delayed. The bones, particularly of the hands, arms, and legs, are involved. Commonly called *soft bone*.

dyscoria. Any abnormality, in form, of the pupil.

dyscrasia. Any abnormal state of the body, as *blood dyscrasia*, a permanent disease of the blood.

dysemesia (*dihss-eh-mee'zee-uh*). Painful vomiting, retching.

dysentery. An inflammation of the large intestine. Characterized by pain, intense diarrhea with passage of small amounts of mucus and blood, and general, serious sickness.

dysfunction. Impairment of function. An example is impairment of eyesight, as in nearsightedness or farsightedness.

dysidrosis (*dihss-ih-droh'sihss*). Any disturbance in the production or excretion of sweat, such as malodorous sweat, too much sweat, too little sweat.

dyskinesia. Impairment of the ability to make any physical motion. An example is the inability to use the hand or fingers after injury to nerves in the arm. Any of the muscles ordinarily under the control of the will may be involved in dyskinesia. The condition may result from a host of diseases.

dysmenorrhea (*dihss-mehn-aw-ree'uh*). Difficult or painful menstruation.

dyspareunia (*dihss-puh-roo'nih-uh*). Difficult or painful sexual intercourse.

dyspepsia. Disturbed digestion. Appears as various combinations of symptoms and is due to various conditions, such as abnormal acidity of the stomach, abnormal flow of bile, inflammation of the stomach, emotional disturbances.

dysphagia (*dihss-fay'jih-uh*). Difficulty in, or inability to, swallow.

dyspnea (*dihsp-nee'uh*). Difficult or labored breathing, as in asthma or heart disease.

dystocia (*dihss-toh'shuh*). Difficult childbirth.

dystrophy (*dihss'truh-fih*). Abnormal development or degeneration. —*adiposogenital d.* Also called *Froehlich's syn-*

drome. Characterized by a female distribution of fat, lack of development of the genitals, and, occasionally, *diabetes insipidus*. Results from an impairment of the pituitary gland and part of the brain that surrounds it. —*dystrophia mediona canaliformis*. Longitudinal grooves in the very center of the fingernail, from the moon to the tip; usually involves the thumb. —*d. myotonica*. An hereditary condition occurring in families. Characterized by a wasting and stiffening of the muscles. It is usually noted early when the infant attempts to use its muscles. —*progressive muscular d*. A wasting disease of muscle characterized by increasing muscular weakness. —*pseudohypertrophic muscular d*. A disorder, beginning in childhood, that occurs in families. Characterized first by unusual growth of the muscles, and later by wasting of the muscles with a forward curvature of the spine, weakness, a waddling walk, inability to rise from the ground, and increasing helplessness. Also called *Erb's dystrophy*.

dysuria (*dihss-you'rih-uh*). Difficult or painful urination.

E

ear. The organ of hearing, consisting of three parts. The *external ear* is composed of a large funnel-shaped outer part known as the *pinna*, and the tube that leads into the skull known as the *external auditory canal*. The *middle ear*, a cavity within the skull, closed off from the outside by the eardrum or tympanum, is crossed by three small bones (the *ossicles*) that are linked together, are somewhat movable, and are attached by the outermost bone to the eardrum and by the innermost bone to the internal ear. Deeper in the skull is the *internal ear*, composed of the *semicircular canals* governing balance and a small bone called the *cochlea* that is filled with fluid and contains a group of specialized nerve cells (the *Organ of Corti*). A small oval aperture in the cochlea is covered with a thin tissue, and this tissue is the drum to which the innermost ossicle or bone of the middle ear is attached. Sound, an air vibration, finally reaches the fluid in the cochlea; the resulting disturbance is transmitted to the Organ of Corti, transformed into appropriate nervous impulses, and communicated through the *acoustic nerve* to that part of the brain where these nervous impulses are translated into what we hear.

eburnation (*ee-buhr-nay'shuhn*). A marked hardening of teeth or bone caused by certain diseases.

ecbolic. 1. Producing abortion or speeding up the labor of childbirth. 2. Any agent that initiates or speeds childbirth, as ergot.

ecchymosis (*ehk-kih-moh'sihss*). An area of blood in the tissues immediately beneath the skin, characterized by a purple color of the skin that gradually changes to brown, green, and yellow. Example: a "black eye."

ecdemic. Denotes diseases brought into a region from without.

echidnotoxin (*eh-kihd-noh-tahk'sihn*). A constituent of snake venom that causes a severe reaction in humans and has a very powerful effect on the nervous system.

echinococcosis (*ee-kigh-nuh-kahk-koh'sihss*). The infestation, particularly in the liver and lung, with a type of tapeworm, *Echinococcus granulosis*. The eggs of this tapeworm are transmitted to man through dogs. In man, large cysts tend to develop.

echolalia (*ehk-oh-lay'lih-uh*). The meaningless repetition of words spoken by others; seen often in cases of schizophrenia.

eclampsia. A form of convulsion occurring most commonly during or after labor.

ecomania (*eck-oh-may'nih-uh*). A psychosis characterized by a hostile, domineering attitude toward members of the family, and one of humility toward those in authority.

ectasia. The widening in diameter of a tubular vessel, as a blood or bronchial vessel. Example: the fine red veins seen at the angles of the nose in the aged or the alcoholic.

ecthyma (*ehk-thigh'muh*). An inflammation of the skin accompanied by large, flat pimples that rupture and become crusted. The pimples vary in size from an eighth to an inch in diameter and are surrounded by a distinct circular area of redness. They appear usually on the legs and thighs, occur in crops, and persist for an indefinite period.

ectopia. An abnormality in position of a part or an organ, usually appearing at birth. Examples: the heart on the right side of the chest; a misplaced kidney.

ectropion. The turning out of a part, especially an eyelid.

eczema (*ehk'zih-muh*). An inflammation of the skin that itches severely and lasts days or years. Not contagious. Eczema is characterized by various combinatoins of skin swelling with tiny blisters, pimples, or scaling of the skin. In the involved skin area, the color is red and shades off into normal flesh-color in the unaffected parts. The cause of eczema is most often allergy.

edema. An excessive accumulation of fluid in the tissues. Edema may be local, as in hives; or it may be general, as in heart failure where the legs, abdominal wall and back are filled with fluid, and where collections of fluid appear in the abdominal cavity and the chest.

edentate (*ee-dehn'tayt*), **edentulous.** Without teeth.

effusion. 1. The accumulation of fluid in the various spaces of the body such as the joints, the chest, the abdomen, the brain cavity. 2. The fluid accumulated. Such accumulation may result from a number of diseases. The fluid may resemble serum of the blood, fill with pus, and become bloody.

ego. At birth, the individual is a maze of instincts pushing for fulfillment and is only vaguely aware of the outer world or reality. This primitive maze of instincts is known as the *id.* Out of the interaction of reality forces and the primitive instincts arises the *ego*. It exists, therefore, between the outer world and the id, and functions to make the id comply with the demands of the world and also to make the world accommodate to the id. The ego, therefore, is a most important regulating force of the mind attempting to bring harmony between the instincts and reality. Ordinarily it represents reason, sanity, logic.

ejaculatio. Ejaculation of semen. —*e. deficiens.* Absence of ejaculation. —*e. praecox.* Premature ejaculation, where the expulsion of semen occurs well before the act of intercourse is completed. —*e. retardata.* Delay of ejaculation, appearing in emotional disturbances due to anxiety.

ejaculation. The ejection of semen.

ejection. 1. The act of expelling or getting rid of, as of excrement. 2. That which is expelled.

elbow. The point at which the arm and the forearm meet; the bend of the arm.

electrocardiogram. Abbreviated ECG or EKG. The record, made by the electrocardiograph, of the various electrical changes that take place within the heart during its action. Provides important information in the diagnosis and treatment of heart disease.

electrocoagulation. The destruction or hardening of tissues by high-frequency currents. Used to destroy small growths of the skin, for the destruction of tonsils in place of surgery, and to seal bleeding small blood vessels during an operation.

electroencephalogram. A record of the electrical changes in the brain made by the *electroencephalograph* or "brain machine." The process by which this record is made is called *electroencephalography.* The electroencephalogram, abbreviated, EEG, is useful in the diagnosis of various conditions of the brain, such as tumors, epilepsy, injury, and others.

elephantiasis (*ehl-eh-fuhn-tigh'uh-sihss*). A persistent, variably sized enlargement of the tissues immediately beneath the skin due to an obstruction of the lymph vessels by worms.

This is the condition in which the legs and arms become enormous. In the male, the scrotum may enlarge to the size of a watermelon. *See also* FILARIA.

elixir. A sweetened, pleasant-smelling, alcoholic liquid used to camouflage unpleasantly tasting medicines.

emasculation. Castration. Removal of the testes, or of the testes and penis.

embolus. Any bit of matter, foreign to the blood, that gains entrance into the blood stream from the individual's body and is carried by the blood until it lodges in an artery and obstructs it (*embolism*). An embolus may be air that comes into the blood either by needle or through some lung injury; cancerous or other cells that by disease break away from their site; fats that may come from the region of a break in bone; clumps of germs; or a foreign body, as a needle or bullet.

embryo. 1. The early stage of development of a young organism. 2. The product of human conception through the third month of pregnancy.

embryology. The science that deals with the embryo and its development.

embryotomy. Any mutilation of the developed infant in the womb performed to aid in its removal when natural delivery is not possible. Embryotomy may vary from decapitation to the fracture of a bone.

emetic (*eh-meht'ihk*). Any agent that causes vomiting.

emetine (*ehm'eh-teen*). A drug that causes sweating and expectoration. Emetine is used mostly against infection with amebas.

emiction. Urination.

emission. 1. A sending forth. 2. A discharge of semen.

emmenagogue. 1. Stimulating menstruation. 2. Any agent that stimulates the menstrual flow.

emollient. 1. Relaxing, soothing, softening. 2. A substance used externally to soften the skin or internally to soothe an inflamed or irritated surface.

empathy. Understanding and appreciation of another's feelings.

emphysema (*em-fih-see'muh*). A condition in which the minute air spaces within the lung at the ends of the tiny bronchial tubes are increased in size; or where there is an abnormal presence of air or gas in the body tissues. Examples are: —*chronic pulmonary e.* Permanent increase in size of the lung air-cells that results in decreased elasticity of the lung and the impairment of its function. —*subcutaneous e.* Accumulation of air or gas under the skin due to infection with a gas-producing germ, as the gas gangrene germ.

empiric. Based on practical observation and not on scientific reasoning.

empyema. The presence of pus in a cavity, hollow organ, or body-space, such as the gall bladder, sinus, heart-sac, and space between the lungs and chest wall.

emulsion. A product made up of minute globules of one liquid suspended throughout a second liquid. The first liquid is not dissolved in the second but retains its identity in minute form throughout the second liquid. Many prescriptions and patent medicines are emulsions. A common example of normally occurring emulsion is milk, in which the fat globules are distributed through the liquid.

encephalitis. Inflammation of the brain. There are many types caused by germs, especially viruses, that may occur after measles, chicken pox, influenza, and with infantile paralysis; due to poison such as lead, and from other disease or injury involving the brain.

encephalogram. An X-ray of the brain made by *encephalography*. This process consists of withdrawing some of the fluid contained in the brain and replacing it with air. The X-ray outlines the areas containing the air on the film. Abnormalities are thus detectable.

encephalomalacia. Softening of the brain, produced by a deficient blood supply. The symptoms vary according to the part of the brain affected. Not uncommonly follows hardening of the arteries in the brain.

encephalon. The brain.

Endamoeba. A type of single-celled animal parasite that lives in human beings. —*e. coli*. An amoeba that lives in the intestinal tract without producing disease. —*e. gingivalis*. A type found in the mouth, about the gums, and in the tartar of the teeth. —*e. histolytica*. The agent that causes amoebic or tropical dysentery; lives in the liver and intestines.

endemic. A disease that occurs more or less constantly in any locality as ragweed hay fever, endemic in the U.S. east of the Rocky Mountains.

endocarditis. An inflammation of the tissue lining the interior of the heart and its valves. —*acute e.* Of sudden onset and severe symptoms as in cases of rheumatic fever and other infectious diseases. Usually the valves of the heart are involved and give rise to a murmur, difficulty in breathing, rapid pulse, and fever. —*chronic e.* An end condition of the *acute e.*, or a condition in itself brought on by syphilis, alcoholism, gout, rheumatism, hardening of the arteries, and other causes.

endocardium. The tissue lining the inside of the heart.

endocrine. 1. Secreting internally. 2. Any of the glands without ducts, as the pituitary, thyroid, and adrenal, whose hormones are passed directly into the blood stream.

endocrinology. The study of the ductless glands and their secretions.

endocrinopathy. A condition arising from an abnormality in one or more of the ductless glands or their secretions, such as overactive thyroid with goiter.

endometriosis. The presence of the tissue that lines the interior of the womb in abnormal locations, as in the bladder wall, or within the abdominal cavity.

endometrium. The tissue that lines the interior wall of the womb.

endoscope. An instrument, usually a hollow tube, equipped with lights and lenses used for the visual examination of the inside of a body cavity, as the abdominal cavity, or hollow organ through its natural outlet as the stomach or urinary bladder. Examples of endoscopes are the bronchoscope, used to examine the breathing tubes; and the cystoscope, used to examine the bladder.

end pleasure. A term used in psychoanalysis to indicate the pleasure accompanying the height of the sexual act brought about by a relief of the tension built up during and before the act.

enema. A liquid instillation into the rectum for treatment or diagnostic purposes. Examples are instillation of barium into the rectum for X-ray purposes, and instillation of glucose for nutritional purposes.

enervation. Reduction of strength, weakness, lassitude.

engram. The indelible impression which experience makes upon nerve cells, much as the impression sound makes upon a wax disc in producing a phonograph record. Under certain circumstances, it is believed, this experience may be relived by virtue of this impression.

enteric. Relating to the intestines.

enteritis. Any inflammation of the intestine.

enterocolitis. Inflammation of the small and large intestines.

enterostomy. The surgical formation of an artificial opening into the intestine through the abdominal wall. Performed to relieve accumulating pressure within the intestine due to obstructions, such as adhesions, tumors, infections.

entropion. The turning in of the edge of the eyelid so that the lashes rub against the eyeball. May occur as a result of diseases that cause scars in the lid; or to spasm of the muscle in the lid.

enucleate (*ih-noo'klih-ayt*). To remove a tumor or an organ in its entirety, as removing an eye from its socket.

enuresis (*en-yuh-ree'sihss*). Inability to control urination. Bed wetting.

enzyme. A substance formed by living cells which, although not partaking in a chemical reaction, promotes its speed. Each enzyme accelerates a specific reaction. One will break starch down to simpler forms as glucose and maltose; another will break off carbon dioxide from organic acids. Enzymes are fundamental to life and upon them depend the direction of the major chemistry of the body.

eosinophil. A type of white blood cell normally found in the blood stream that has an affinity for a red-staining dye known as *eosin*. Under the microscope such white cells show many red grains within them.

eosinophilia. An increase beyond normal in the number of eosinophils in the blood stream or in tissues. Commonly occurs in allergy, infestation with worms, and other conditions.

epicanthus. An abnormality existing at birth and continuing through life in which a fold of skin covers the inner angle of the eye. The resulting slant is called epicanthus. This is a racial characteristic of the Mongolian. It is not uncommon in infants of other races in whom the bone of the nose is underdeveloped.

epicranium. The structures covering the top of the skull; the scalp, made up of tough fibrous tissue, muscle, hair.

epidemic. An unusual prevalence of a disease affecting large numbers of people over a wide area.

epidemiology. The study of the occurrence and distribution of disease.

epidermophytid (*ehp-uh-duhr-moh-figh'tihd*). An eruption of the skin, characterized by blisters and scaling, produced by an allergic reaction to a fungus, *Epidermophyton*. Example: the scaling of palms and fingers often seen in golfers due to an allergic reaction to athlete's foot.

epidermophytosis. A general name used to include any fungus infection of the feet producing blisters, scaliness, and itching, such as athlete's foot.

epididymectomy (*eh-puh-dihd-ih-mehk'tuh-mih*). The surgical removal of the *epididymis*, a part of the tube system through which semen passes from the testes into the urethra. The epididymis lies behind and at the upper pole of the testis and is connected to it by many fine ducts.

epididymis. *See* EPIDIDYMECTOMY.

epididymitis (*eh-pih-dihd-ih-migh'tihss*). Inflammation of the epididymis, often as the result of gonorrhea.

epiglottis. A small elastic piece of gristle covered by moist thin tissue that forms a lid for the voice box and that closes on swallowing to prevent food from going into the voice box and to help direct food into the gullet.

epilation. The removal of hair by the root by chemical means, X-ray, or plucking.

epilepsy. A nervous system condition manifesting episodes of unconsciousness with or without convulsions. There are many types of epilepsy. The most common are: *Grand-mal.* Characterized by sudden loss of consciousness, stiffening of the body, bluing of the skin, spasm of all the muscles with the eyes turned up, frothing at the mouth, and, frequently, passage of urine, confusion, deep sleep, awakening with no memory of the episode; *Petit-mal.* Characterized by very short lapses into unconsciousness that may appear as a sudden momentary pause in movement or conversation, rarely lasting 30 seconds (frequent in children; may occur as often as 200 times a day; the patient here rarely falls or has muscular spasm); *Jacksonian e.* Spasms of muscles occurring in attacks but localized to one side of the body, or one area of muscles often without loss of consciousness in the beginning, but as the disease progresses the spasms may become general.

epileptoid. Resembling epilepsy.

epiphora. A continuous overflow of tears due to unusual tear production or an obstruction in the tear duct.

episcleritis. An inflammation of the tissues underneath the lining tissue of the white of the eye; or inflammation of the white of the eye itself.

episiotomy. Cutting of the wall of the vagina during childbirth to avoid undue tearing.

epispadias (*ehp-uh-spay'dih-uhss*). A condition in which the opening of the penis is on its upper surface.

epistaxis. Nosebleed.

epithelioma (*ehp-uh-thee-lih-oh'muh*). A tumor, not malignant, that arises from a type of tissue known as *epithelium*. This tissue is of the general type that forms the skin and lines all the hollow organs, such as the stomach, womb, bladder and all the passages of the respiratory tract.

epithelization. The growth of epithelium over a raw surface, as the regrowth of skin over a small cut.

epizoic. An animal parasite living on the surface of the body, such as the louse.

erection. The enlargement, when engorged with blood, of certain organs made up of elastic tissue and containing large blood spaces, as the penis or clitoris.

ergophobia. Morbid dread of work.

ergot (*ehr'guht*). A drug made from a fungus that grows on cereal plants, as rye. In medieval times breads made from infested crops produced epidemics of a condition then called St. Anthony's fire. Ergot causes powerful spasms of the womb and is used medically in checking unusual monthly bleeding or the bleeding following childbirth. It is not infrequently used to induce abortion. This procedure is dangerous since it may lead to poisoning and eventually to gangrene of the extremities.

ergotism. Poisoning with ergot. May result in spasms and painful contractions of the muscles, or in complete closure of small blood vessels with resulting gangrene because of lack of blood supply.

erosion. Destruction of the surface of an area by inflammation or injury. Commonly seen on the neck of the womb as the result of old birth injuries or local infection.

erotogenic (*ih-roh-toh-jehn'ihk*). Causing or originating from sexual desire or passion.

erotogenic zones. Sensitive areas of the body, stimulation of which gives rise to sexual feelings. There are many of these, the three major ones being the lips and mouth, the anus, and the genitals.

erotomania. A morbid exaggeration of affection toward the opposite sex.

eructation. Belching.

erysipelas (*ehr-uh-sihp'uh-luhss*). An infectious disease characterized by inflammation of the skin and the underlying tissue that spreads from area to area caused by a germ, *Streptococcus pyogenes*. Sulfa drugs are very effective in the treatment.

erysipeloid. An infection that occurs on the hands of people who handle infected fish or meat. There are many circumscribed red eruptions due to a germ, *Erysipellthrix rhusiopathiae*.

erythema (*ehr-uh-thee'muh*). A redness of the skin that usually occurs in irregular shapes and varying sizes. There are many kinds of erythema, some of which are serious. Examples: sunburn, or the redness that surrounds hives.

erythema polyneuropathy. A disease of unknown cause frequently seen in children in the last quarter of their first year. It is characterized by itchy, swollen, dark pink hands and feet, marked sweating, light sensitiveness, lack of appetite, insomnia, and irritability. Ordinarily, the disease lasts several months and the patient recovers. Also called *Feer's disease, Selter's disease, pink disease, acrodynia*.

erythrocyte (*ih-rihth'roh-sight*). A red blood cell.

erythroderma. A disturbance of the skin characterized by abnormal redness; also called erythema.

erythromelalgia (*ih-rith-roh-muh-laal'jih-uh*). A condition of unknown cause, usually affecting the feet, less commonly the hands. Characterized by mottling of the skin, redness, pain, and increase in the skin temperature.

eschar. The sloughed tissue caused by heat, caustic substances like lye, or corrosive substances like acid.

escharotic. Producing a slough; caustic; any substance that produces an eschar, like lye and acid.

escutcheon. The pattern of hair-growth in the pubic area that differs in the male and in the female. In the female, it is a triangle with the base upward; in the male, it is diamond-shaped with the hair growing onto the abdomen.

esophagitis (*ee-sahf-uh-jigh'tihss*). An inflammation of the gullet.

esophagoscope. A tubular instrument illuminated for direct visualization of the interior of the gullet.

esophagospasm. Muscular spasm of the gullet.

esophagus. The gullet, extending from the throat to the stomach, about nine inches in length, the wall of which is composed of muscle and fibrous tissue.

estrogen. Any substance that is capable of stimulating the various changes in the lining tissue of the womb ordinarily under control of the ovaries, as those that accompany the menstrual cycle.

estrus. All of the changes in the lining tissue of the womb that accompany menstruation.

etherization. Administration of ether to cause anesthesia.

ethmoid. A bone at the base and the front of the skull that has many holes through which the nerve of smell passes; the bone that forms the upper part of the nose.

ethmoidectomy. The surgical removal of parts of the ethmoid bone or the air cells in the ethmoid bone that constitute the *ethmoid sinuses*.

ethmoiditis. Inflammation of the ethmoid sinuses or the ethmoid bone.

etiology. The study of the causes of diseases.

eunuch (*you'nuhk*). A male whose testes or testes and penis have been removed.

eunuchoidism (*you-nuh-koy'dihzm*). A condition in which the testes are present but inactive.

euphonia. A normal, clear condition of the voice.

euphoria. An exaggerated sense of well-being.

Eustachian (*you-stay'shuhn*). Pertaining to the auditory tube, that leads from the middle ear to an area just behind the tonsils in the throat.

euthanasia (*you-thuh-nay'zhuh*). The painless putting to death of those who are suffering from incurable and painful disease.

evacuant. A medicine that empties an organ, especially the bowel, as Epsom salts.

evagination. Out-pouching. Turning inside out, as the turning inside out of a finger of a glove.

eversion. An outward turning, as the folding of the upper lid upon itself for the purpose of removing a cinder.

evisceration (*ih-vihss-suhr-ay'shuhn*). Literally to disembowel; burst belly; the protrusion of the abdominal organs through an abdominal incision after an operation.

exacerbation. An increase in the degree of sickness.

exanthema (*ehk-saan-thee'muh*). A fever with eruption, as measles, chicken pox, and other contagious diseases.

excoriation. The wearing or rubbing away of a portion of the skin by disease or injury.

excrescence. An abnormal out-growth upon the body such as a wart or tumor, or the cauliflower ear of boxers.

exostosis. A bony out-growth from the surface of a bone.

expectorant. A remedy that stimulates expectoration. Any medicine that helps bring up phlegm.

extern. A medical school student or graduate who helps in a hospital but lives outside of it.

extirpation. The complete surgical removal or destruction of a part.

extrasystole (*ehks-truh-sihss'tuh-lee*). A heartbeat that occurs before its normal time in the rhythm of the heart, and that is followed by a pause delaying the succeeding heartbeat. The patient may or may not be aware of it. When he is, he may feel his heart "stand still," or may feel a particularly forceful heartbeat.

extravasation. 1. The passing of body fluid from its proper place into the surrounding tissue, as blood from a ruptured vessel into the skin after an injury, or urine into the surrounding tissue after rupture of the bladder. 2. The liquid so passed.

extremity. The terminal or far end of any part as the *lower e.*: the hip, thigh, leg, ankle, and foot; or the *upper e.*: the shoulder, arm, forearm, wrist, and hand.

exudate (*eks'you-dayt*). The material that passes through the unbroken walls of a blood vessel into the surrounding tissue, as pus, in inflammation.

eyeground. The internal aspect of the eye as seen through the pupil by use of an ophthalmoscope.

F

facies (*fay'shih-eez*). The appearance of the face, as the adenoid facies, resulting from adenoids that interfere with breathing through the nose, characterized by a thin narrow nose, open mouth, and somewhat stupid appearance.

far point. The most distant point that an eye can see distinctly when completely relaxed.

fascia (*faash'ih-uh*). The fibrous tissue that lies under the skin, or between muscles forming sheaths through which the muscles run, or surrounding other internal structures, as nerves and blood vessels.

fatigue. Exhaustion of strength; weariness from exertion; a condition in which, because of previous overactivity, the power or capacity to respond to stimulation is diminished or lost. The word is used loosely to mean an emotional illness, as in *battle f.*, shell shock; *flying f.*, occurring in flyers; *operational f.*, occurring in combat flying.

fauces (*faw'seez*). A space in the back part of the mouth, surrounded by the soft palate, the tonsil arches, and the base of the tongue.

favism. A disease common in Sicily and Sardinia characterized by severe anemia due to sensitivity to the broad bean. Favism results from eating the seeds or from inhalation of the pollen of the bean.

favus (*fay'vuhs*). A skin disease due to the fungus, *Tricho-phyton*, characterized by cup-shaped crusts, round, sulphur yellow in color, that have a mousy odor. The scalp is most commonly affected but the disease may occur elsewhere on the skin.

fear reaction. A popular name for an emotional illness, particularly one developed in combat, in which anxiety is shown by the conscious fear of a particular event or object.

feces (*fee'seez*). The excretions of the bowels composed of unabsorbed food, indigestible matter, and intestinal secretion.

fecundity. The potential reproductive capacity of the individual.

fee splitting. An unethical division of the consultant's fee between the referring physician and himself.

fellatio (*feh-lay'shih-oh*). A form of sexual perversion in which the male genital is placed in the mouth of another.

fellator. A male receiver in the practice of fellatio.

fellatrice (*feh-luh-trihss'*). A female who practices fellatio.

felon. An infection which is deep under the skin, on the far end and inner surface of a finger.

femur (*fee'muhr*). The thighbone.

fenestration. The presence of small openings in any structure. Losely used to designate a special operation, *Lempert's operation*, to relieve deafness in certain specific cases.

fermentation. The decomposition of complex substances under the influence of enzymes. Example: the production of alcohol from cereal through the agency of yeast.

fester. To produce pus.

feticide (*fee'tih-sighd*). The killing of the developing infant in the womb, usually intentional, to produce an abortion.

fetish. Anything which becomes unusually attractive because of its association with sexual pleasure. Such association is made unconsciously. Examples: hair, shoes, articles of clothing.

fetus (*fee'tuhss*). The unborn offspring from the end of the third month until birth. Before this period (conception to the third month) the proper term is *embryo*.

fever. The increase of body temperature above normal, in humans above 98.6° Fahrenheit.

fiber. A threadlike structure, as nerve fiber, muscle fiber.

fibrillation. A quivering of muscle fibers. Sometimes seen in the calf muscle. —*cardiac f.* A quivering of the heart muscles that through disease have fallen out of their normal rhythmic action. When this occurs in the ventricles, the large chambers of the heart, it is almost always fatal.

fibrin (*figh'brihn*). A protein substance that is produced by elements of the blood and tissues and forms a network as the base of clots.

fibroid. A tumor of the womb consisting of tough, fibrous tissue.

fibroidectomy. The surgical removal of a fibroid of the womb.

fibroma. A tumor, not ordinarily serious, composed principally of tough, fibrous tissue.

fibrosis. The growth of tough, fibrous tissue in an organ or part beyond the amount naturally present.

fibula (*fihb'yuh-luh*). The slender bone at the outer part of the leg that lies parallel to the shinbone, and with the shinbone comprises the bony structure of the leg.

filament. A small, threadlike structure, as the tail of a sperm.

filaria (*fih-laa'rih-uh*). A long, threadlike worm that lives in the blood or lymph vessels, and at times in the tissues and cavities of the infested human being. The small growing forms or *microfilariae* are found in the blood stream and lymph from which they are taken up by any one of a number of blood-sucking insects. Within the insect body the young form grows into adulthood and is passed on to the other animals or to humans by the insect's bite. Commonly the cause of *elephantiasis*. *See also* ELEPHANTIASIS.

filariasis (*fih-luh-righ'uh-sihss*). The state of being infested with filaria.

finger. A digit of the hand. —*baseball f.* A dislocation, by a baseball injury, of the last joint of a finger with rupture of part of that tendon that opens out the finger, causing the last segment of the finger to hang losely. —*clubbed f.* A finger in which the end segment is short and broad, resembling the bulbous end of a club. Occurs as the result of prolonged interference with breathing as in certain lung and heart diseases. Also called *chronic hypertrophic pulmonary osteoarthropathy*, *drumstick f.*, *Hippocratic f.* —*hammer f.* A deformity in which the middle segment of a finger is bent toward the palm. Present at birth.

finger cot. A small sheath of rubber or other material for protection of the finger when it is injured and dressed, or to prevent infection of the examiner's finger when doing a rectal examination. Also called *finger stall*.

fissure. A groove or cleft. Fissures are normal in various parts of the anatomy, as in the skull, the brain, the liver; and abnormal, as cracks in the skin or longitudinal ulcers in lining tissues. An example is a rectal fissure, i.e., a long ulceration of the lining membrane of the rectum often associated with piles.

fistula (*fihss'choo-luh*). A narrow tube or a canal, the result of incomplete healing of a wound, an abscess or other disease condition, or an imperfect development in growth. Ordinarily the fistula contains and discharges fluid, either pus or the contents of an organ or cavity of the body. Fistulas that open from an organ to the exterior of the body are named according to the organ involved as *stomach f.*, *intestinal f.*, *bladder f.* When the fistula connects two organs, the names of both organs are applied to the fistula, for example *vesico-*

vaginal f., where the urinary bladder and the vagina are connected by such a canal.

fistulectomy (*fihss-chuh-lehk'tuh-mih*). The surgical excision of a fistula.

flagellate. A microscopic single-celled animal furnished with a slender, whip-like extension that is involved in propelling the organism.

flagellation. 1. To flog or beat. 2. Whipping or beating as a means of producing sexual gratification.

flank. The fleshy part between the ribs and the hip; the outer side of the buttock, hip, and thigh.

flatfoot. *Pes planus.* A defect existing from birth or acquired as a result of loss of the normal muscle tension in the foot caused by long standing, bad walking, ill-fitting shoes. The normal arch in the sole of the foot drops.

flatulence. The presence of gas in stomach and intestines.

flatus (*flay'tuhss*). Gas, especially air or gas in the stomach and intestines. —*f. vaginalis.* The expulsion of gas from the vagina accompanying intercourse due to the introduction of air into the vaginal canal.

flexion. Bending; the state of being bent.

flexor. A muscle that bends or flexes a limb or a part, as the large muscle of the upper arm or the biceps that acts to bend the elbow and draw up the forearm.

flight of ideas. A rapid barrage of ideas and fancies that follow one upon another through the mind, usually accompanying acute mania, a form of insanity.

floating. Unusual movability or position of a structure due to stretching or destruction of its natural attachment, or to some deficiency in the structure. —*f. kidney.* A kidney displaced from its normal immovable position that, because of its abnormal motion, may cause trouble by bending the tubular passage, *ureter*, to the bladder.

florid. Of a bright red color, as the florid complexion often seen in persons with high blood pressure, or in the chronic alcoholic.

fluoroscope. An X-ray instrument used to see into the body. Thus the form and motion of internal structures can be detected.

flush. 1. To blush; become filled with blood due to widening of the small blood vessels in, and just under, the skin. Flush occurs in emotional states, overactivity of the thyroid, inflammation, fever, and chronic malnutrition. 2. To clean a cavity or a wound with a stream of water.

flutter. Irregular, quick motion; agitation. *—atrial f.* An irregularity in the beating of the heart when the small chambers of the heart (*atria*) beat with much greater rapidity than the larger chambers of the heart (*ventricles*). The ratio of speed of atria to ventricles may be two to one, three to one, four to one.

flux. An unusually great flow of any of the body excretions, especially the bowel contents.

folliculitis (*fuh-lihk-yuh-ligh'tihss*). Inflammation of a group of follicles (small cavities or sacs that secrete a fluid), as the hair follicles which produce oil. *—f. barbae.* "Barber's itch." Inflammation of the hair follicles of the beard. Also called *sycosis. —f. decalvans.* Inflammation of the hair follicles resulting in patches of baldness.

fomentation. 1. The application of wet heat to relieve inflammation and pain. 2. The substance used to convey heat and moisture, as hot boric acid, Epsom salts.

fontanel (*fahn-tuh-nehll'*). A space between the bones of the skull before birth and in infancy that closes in the course of normal bone development. There are many fontanels, the most obvious being the *anterior f.*, a diamond-shaped space in the middle and forward part of the skull just behind the hairline; the *posterior f.*, a triangular space in the back of the middle of the base of the skull.

foramen (*faw-ray'muhn*). An opening or perforation, particularly in a bone. There are many of these in the body named according to the area in which they occur or by their shape. Example: the *f. magnum*, a large, oval hole in the center and lower part of the base of the skull through which passes the spinal cord and its veins, arteries, and accessory nerves.

forensic. Pertaining to a law court, as forensic medicine that deals with various aspects of medicine related to the law; crimes of violence; poisonings; the determination of suicide or homicide.

forepleasure. The physical and emotional erotic experience that is accompanied by an increase in urgency preceding the climax of the sexual act.

fornication. Sexual intercourse of persons not married to each other.

fracture. The break or breaking of bone or gristle. —*chip. f.* The breaking off of a tiny fragment of bone. —*Colles' f.* A common type of wrist fracture in which the displaced parts give the hand and wrist the appearance of a fork, lying with curve up. —*greenstick f.* An incomplete break in one of the long bones, as the arm or thigh bone. Commonly seen in children where the bone is bent and splintered only on the hump of the bend.

fragilitas (*fruh-jihl'lih-tuhs*). Brittleness. —*f. crinium.* A wasting condition of the hair where the individual hairs split, break into numerous longitudinal parts, or break off. —*f. ossium.* A disease of the long bones, as the arm and thighbone, characterized by unusual brittleness and episodes of many breaks associated with a blue cast to the whites of the eyes. This disease occurs in families. Also called *Lobstein's disease, Eddowe's disease.*

fragility. The characteristic of being easily destroyed and broken. —*capillary f.* Weakness of the capillaries, the smallest diameter blood vessels, as in a disease called *purpura,* leading to the recurrent rupture of these vessels and the appearance of large black and blue spots all over the body.

frenulum (*frehn'yuh-luhm*). A small frenum. —*f. of the clitoris.* Two folds of lining tissue arising from the vaginal lips and united under the tip of the clitoris, thus checking its movements. —*f. of the tongue.* The fold of lining tissue under the tongue easily seen in the mirror by opening the mouth and placing the tip of the tongue as far back as possible on the roof of the mouth.

frenum (*free'nuhm*). A fold of skin or lining tissue that checks or limits the movement of any organ.

frigidity. The absence of sexual desire in women, usually of psychological origin; coldness.

frontal. 1. Relating to the front part of the body or an organ. 2. Relating to the forehead.

frostbite. A condition produced by long exposure to severe cold. The result is similar to that caused by burns. There are three stages: redness, blistering, and sloughing. The parts most commonly affected are the fingers, toes, tip of the nose, and ears.

frottage (*fraw-tahj'*). 1. Rubbing, massage. 2. A form of sexual activity brought on by the proximity of two bodies.

frustration. The denial of gratification or the thwarting of an instinctual drive.

fulguration (*fuhl-gyuh-ray'shuhn*). The destruction of tissues by means of electric sparks. Often used on cancerous tumors, and instead of the knife for destruction of the tonsils.

fulminant. Relating to a disease that comes on suddenly with great severity and is very rapid in course.

function. The normal and specific action of a part.

fundament. 1. The base or foundation. 2. The seat, as the buttocks.

fundus. The base of an organ or the part farthest from the opening of the organ. —*f. oculi.* The back part of the inside of the eye. —*f. uteri.* The part of the womb farthest from its neck.

fungicide. An agent that kills fungi.

fungoid. Looking like a fungus.

fungus. A very low form of plant life; mold.

funiculitis. Inflammation of the cord that suspends the testes in the scrotum, the *spermatic cord.*

funny bone. The outer aspect of the elbow that is crossed by part of the ulnar nerve. Blows in this area result in a painful, tingling sensation in the hand.

furuncle (*fyou'ruhn-kuhl*). A boil, usually the result of an infection of a hair follicle, occasionally due to the spread of germs through the blood stream.

furunculosis. A condition of numerous or successive crops of boils.

fusiform (*fyou'zuh-fawrm*). Spindle-shaped.

fusion. Melting together, uniting. —*spinal f.* The union of two or more vertebrae thus immobilizing part of the spine. May occur as a result of disease. Usually designates a surgical procedure, for the treatment of spinal deformities, severe arthritis, or tuberculosis of the spine.

G

gait. The manner of walking. —*ataxic g.* Walking with deficient control of the extent of motion of leg and foot. The foot is raised higher than ordinary, thrown forward, and brought down suddenly on its entire sole. —*cerebellar g.* A zigzagging walk that resembles the staggering of an alcoholic accentuated by sudden lurching.

galactischia (*guh-laak-tihss'kih-uh*). The suppression of the secretion of milk.

galactorrhea (*guh-laak-tuh-ree'uh*). An excessive flowing of milk.

galeophobia (*gay-lih-oh-foh'bih-uh*). A morbid fear of cats.

gall bladder. A pear-shaped sac on the under surface of the right half of the liver. Its function is to store and concentrate bile, and to secrete mucus. Stones may form in the gall bladder from the various elements composing the bile. They may cause no symptoms for a long time. However, if a stone moves into the narrow end of the gall bladder or into the duct system leading from it, pain will result. The pain is severe and cramping and often shoots into the collar bone and shoulder blade regions. Nausea, vomiting, slight fever, jaundice, and light-colored stools may accompany this pain. Such attacks usually subside in a few hours, with the stone falling back into the gall bladder proper or passing through the duct system into the small intestine. Repeated attacks may result in acute inflammation of the gall bladder (acute cholecystitis), the symptoms of which are similar to those just described, but the fever is more marked and the pain may require repeated doses of opiates.

ganglion. 1. A collection of nerve cells outside the brain or spinal cord that serves as a relay station for impulses transmitted from or to the nerves. 2. A fluid-containing sac in a tendon or a joint that often appears in the tendons of the back of the hand or wrist as a lump that gradually increases in size. Treatment: rupturing with a sharp blow.

gangrene. 1. The death of a part of the body due to failure of blood supply to that part as the result of disease or injury. 2. The decay that occurs in dead tissue. Causes other than injury are hardening of the arteries, diabetes, blood clots, ergot poisoning, and many similar conditions.

gastralgia (*gaas-traal'jih-uh*). Pain in the stomach.

gastrectomy. The surgical removal of part, or all, of the stomach.

gastric. Relating to the stomach.

gastritis. Inflammation of the stomach. There are many forms, each a result of poisoning by mouth, infection, or allergy.

gastrocnemius (*gaas-trohk-nee'mih-uhss*). The large muscle in the back of the leg that comprises almost the entire calf.

gastroenteritis. Inflammation of the stomach and intestine.
gastroenterologist. A specialist in diseases of the stomach and intestines. One who practices gastroenterology.
gastroenterostomy. The surgical formation of a communication between the stomach and the small intestine, performed in cases of stomach ulcer in order to short-circuit the food around the ulcer.
gastrojejunostomy. The surgical formation of a communication between the front part of the stomach and the second division of the small intestine, performed commonly in cases of peptic ulcer.
gastrorrhagia (*gaas-troh-ray'jih-uh*). Hemorrhage from the stomach.
gavage (*gah-vahzh'*). Giving liquid nourishment through a tube inserted into the mouth, down the gullet, and into the stomach.
gelotolepsy (*jehl'uh-tuh-lehp-sih*). A sudden loss of the normal muscle tension; a sudden attack of flaccidity of the entire body accompanied by a short loss of consciousness during laughter.
genesis. The origin of anything; the development of a specific thing or type. Often used as a combining form in medicine to indicate this meaning, as *carcinogenesis*, the origin or development of cancer.
genicular (*jeh-nihk'yuh-luhr*). Relating to the knee joint, as the genicular vein of the knee.
genital. Relating to the sex organs or the organs of reproduction.
genitalia. The organs of generation. The male has two testes with their ducts, the prostate gland, the penis, and the urethra. The female has the vaginal lips, the vaginal canal, the ovaries, the Fallopian tubes, and the womb.
genitourinary. Relating to the genitalia and the organs of urine formation and excretion (kidneys, ureters, bladder, urethra).

genu (*jee'nyou*). 1. The knee. 2. Any structure like the knee, i.e., any structure that bends like the knee.

geriatrician (*jehr-ih-uh-trihsh'uhn*). A specialist in the treatment of diseases of old age. Also called *geriatrist*.

geriatrics (*jehr-ih-aat'rihks*). The branch of medicine concerned with old age and its diseases.

German measles. *See* RUBELLA.

germicide. Any agent that destroys germs.

gerontology (*jehr-ahn-tahl'uh-jih*). The scientific study of old age.

gestation. Pregnancy.

Giardia (*jih-ahr'dih-uh*). A type of microscopic single-celled animal parasite. —*g. lamblia*. A species of giardia found in the small intestine of man (doubtful whether it causes disease).

giardiasis (*jih-ahr-digh'uh-sihss*). The presence of *Giardia lamblia* in the small intestine of man.

gibbous (*gihb'uhss*). Humpbacked, particularly on one side.

gigantism (*jigh'gaan-tihsm*). Unusual height and size. A height in man over seventy-nine inches due to an oversupply of hormone from a part of the pituitary gland. Gigantism may be of three types: 1. *Normal*, in which the body proportions and sex functions are normal. 2. *Eunuchoid*, where female physical characteristics are present, such as female distribution of fat, and sexual deficiency. 3. *Acromegalic*, in which characteristics of acromegaly are present.

gingiva (*jihn-jigh'vuh*). Generally, the gums. Specifically, the gum that surrounds the tooth.

gingivitis (*jin-jih-vigh'tihss*). Inflammation of the gums.

gland. A cell, tissue, or organ that manufactures and expels a substance that is used elsewhere in the body (secretion), or that is eliminated from the body (excretion). Examples of glands that secrete are the adrenal, the thyroid, the pituitary. Examples of glands that excrete are, the oil glands of the skin and the salivary gland.

glans. The cone-shaped body that forms the tip of the penis (*glans penis*) or the tip of the clitoris (*glans clitoridis*).

glaucoma. An eye disease that is characterized by greater than normal pressure within the eyeball. This increased pressure results in an unusual hardness of the eyeball that can be detected by feel; a depression of the head of the optic nerve; a narrowing of the field of vision; lack of sensation in the transparent front part of the eye; a colored halo seen around artificial lights; a decrease in sight that may eventually lead to blindness. There are many types of glaucoma, all primarily due to a lack of drainage of the fluid from within the eyeball.

gleet. A late stage of inflammation of the canal within the penis, characterized by a slight, pus-laden discharge from the penis. Frequently the late stage of gonorrhea.

glioma (*gligh-oh'muh*). A tumor consisting of supporting tissue of the nervous system that appears chiefly in the nerves themselves, the spinal cord, the brain, and the adrenal glands.

globule. A small, spherical droplet of liquid or semi-liquid material, as the *milk globule*, a fat drop in milk.

globulin. A class of proteins found in living matter; an important part of human blood. Three fractions are known: The *alpha g.* contains enzymes and hormones; the *beta g.* contains the elements important in determining the blood group of the individual and also certain elements involved in blood clotting; the *gamma g.* contains most of the protective substances known as antibodies.

globus (*gloh'buhss*). A ball or sphere. —*g. hystericus.* "Lump in the throat"; the choking sensation seen frequently in hysteria.

glomerulonephritis (*gloh-muhr-you-loh-nih-frigh'tihss*). A kidney disease almost always preceded by or associated with an infection, particularly one caused by a streptococcus. In the course of the disease, high blood pressure, convulsions, dropsy, and death may occur.

glomerulus (*gloh-mehr'you-luhss*). 1. A small round mass.

2. An important element of the kidney. The kidney is composed of individual units known as *renal corpuscles*. The renal corpuscle is a sphere or near-sphere, microscopic in size, hollowed at one end. The glomerulus is a tuft of small blood-vessel loops that projects into the hollow of the corpuscle, much as the fist into the cupped palm.

glossa. The tongue.

glossalgia (*glaw-saal'jih-uh*). Pain in the tongue.

glossectomy. The surgical removal of the tongue.

glossitis. Inflammation of the tongue.

glossodynia (*glahs-oh-dihn'ih-uh*). Pain in the tongue.

glossopyrosis (*glahs-oh-pigh-roh'sihss*). A burning sensation in the tongue.

glossotrichia (*glaw-soh-trihk'ih-uh*). Hairy tongue. Seen in some cases of disease caused by a deficiency of vitamins.

glottis. The space between the vocal cords.

glucose. A colorless, or yellowish, thick sweet liquid that dissolves readily in water. Glucose is a simple sugar that is obtained from the more complex sugars, as cane sugar. Liquid glucose is used for its food value when given by vein, and its effect is to withdraw fluid from the body tissues and increase urination. Glucose is a normal constituent of the blood stream, but when present in higher than normal values in the blood *diabetes mellitus* must be suspected.

gluten. A mixture of proteins found in cereals, as wheat, rye, barley. Gluten gives toughness to dough.

glycosuria (*gligh-koh-soo'ree-uh*). The presence of sugar in the urine. —*alimentary g*. The result of eating an excessive amount of carbohydrates. —*anxiety g*. The result of worry, usually of very short duration. —*artificial g*. When a certain part of the brain stem is injured, sugar appears in the urine. This is a common laboratory procedure in animals. —*diabetic g*. Due to *diabetes mellitus*. —*renal g*. A condition, caused by some defect of development, in which the threshold for sugar is low. Unlike diabetes, where sugar appears in the urine only after the blood sugar rises to a considerable height above normal, sugar will appear in the urine in *renal g.* when the sugar in the blood is at a normal level. The condition has little significance and is no cause for concern. —*toxic g.* Sugar in the urine after poisoning with morphine, curare, chloral, chloroform, or carbon monoxide.

glycyrrhyza (*glih-sih-righ'zuh*). Licorice. Extracts of this material are mixed with drugs in various medicines.

gnathic (*naa'thihk*). Relating to the jaw.

goiter. An increase in size of the thyroid gland that lies in the lower part of the neck, in front of the windpipe, like an "H" with the crossbar being very small and the two vertical bars being wide and heavy. There are many types of goiter, in some of which the gland is generally enlarged or *diffuse*, and in others enlarged in part or in small tumor-like masses, when it is called *cystic*. A common variety, known as "ingrown goiter" or *exophthalmic g.*, is caused by excessive manufacture of thyroid hormone by the gland. Exophthalmic g. is characterized by some enlargement of the gland, nervousness, tremor of the hands and tongue, protrusion of the eyes, weakness, and loss of weight. If unchecked, this condition may lead to death. Also called *Graves' disease, hyperthyroidism, thyrotoxicosis, toxic goiter.*

goitrogenic (*goy-troh-jeh'nihk*). Producing goiter, as diets deficient in iodine; or some of the newer drugs that tend to relieve hyperthyroidism, as thiouracil.

gonad. A general term for the ovary or testes.

gonadotrophin. A hormone that stimulates the ovary or testes. It is obtained from the pituitary gland, the urine of pregnant women, or the blood of pregnant horses.

gonococcus (*gahn-uh-kahk'uhs*). The common name for the germ causing gonorrhea. Its scientific name is *Neisseria gonorrheae.*

gonorrhea (*gahn-uh-ree'uh*). An infection contracted by intimate contact with another human being, characterized by an inflammation of the lining membrane of the urethra and the cavities that are near it, accompanied by pain, burning on urination, and a copious discharge of pus. The complications that may follow are inflammation of the prostate, abscesses about the urethra, inflammation of the bladder, and inflammation of the eyes. Gonorrhea may also cause arthritis, inflammation of the lining of the heart, and inflammation of the ovarian tubes.

gout. A condition in which there is a decrease in the excretion of one of the end products of food breakdown, *uric acid*. Gout is characterized by attacks of acute, painful arthritis usually involving one joint, most often the great toe. The joint is ordinarily hot, tender, red with shiny surrounding skin. Fever appears. Between attacks there is complete freedom from symptoms. After many attacks a permanent deformity of the joint may occur. Often the kidney becomes involved following prolonged gout. A common associated condition is the deposit of small, hard, chalk-like masses, called *tophi*, in the skin about the fingernails, or the ear, and in the gristle of the joints.

graft. A piece of tissue such as skin or bone to replace a defect in the body; an entire cornea to replace a defective one.

granulation. Minute red particles or masses that are grossly visible at the bottom of a wound during its healing process. These tiny masses consist of newly formed capillaries and cells that eventually form scar tissue or "proud flesh."

granulocyte (*graan'yuh-luh-sight*). A full-grown white blood cell. Within its protoplasm are tiny rounded masses called granules. Granules are of three varieties depending upon the kind of dye stains for which the granules have an affinity: *eosinophilic*, those that stain red with *eosin*, an acid dye; *basophilic*, those that stain blue with an alkaline dye; or *neutrophilic*, those that stain with a neutral dye. The granulocyte is named according to the type of granule it has, *eosinophilic g., basophilic g., neutrophilic g.*

granuloma (*graan-yuh-loh'muh*). A visible mass of inflammatory tissue in which the process of granule formation is apparent. There are many varieties of granuloma due to various infections, such as syphilis, yaws and other venereal infections, and also at times due to noninfectious malignant diseases.

gravel. A sandlike material that makes up kidney or bladder stones, and that is often passed in the urine.

gravid. Pregnant.

groin. The depression between the thigh and the abdomen.

gumma. A result of late syphilis, that can occur almost anywhere in the body but is seen particularly in the heart, liver, and brain. Gumma is an easily observed mass up to an inch in diameter, with a firm rubber consistency and a decaying center.

gustation. The act of tasting; the sense of taste.

gustatory (*guhss'tuh-taw-rih*). Relating to the sense of taste.

gynandromorphism (*jihn-aan-droh-mawr'fihsm*). A condition in which the individual has characteristic tissues of both male and female. Example: a male with well-developed breasts and an incomplete scrotum that may contain the beginnings of a vagina.

gynatresia (*jihn-uh-tree'zhuh*). The condition in which there is no passageway in the vagina.

gynecoid (*jihn'uh-koyd*). Like or resembling a woman.

gynecologist. A specialist in the diseases of women, especially those affecting the sexual organs. One who practices gynecology.

gynecology (*jihn-uh* (or *gigh-nuh*)-*kahl'uh-jih*). The science of women's diseases, especially those affecting the sexual organs.

gynecomastia (*jihn-uh-koh-maas'tih-uh*). Enlargement of the breast in the male, usually one-sided. Gynecomastia may accompany diseases of the ductless glands, especially of the testes and the adrenals, may follow various malignant tumors, may result from the use of certain hormones, or may have no apparent cause, often coming on in adolescence.

gynoplasty (*jigh'noh-plaass-tih*). Plastic surgery of the female genitals.

H

hallucination. The perception of objects and sensations that have no reality and no external causes.

hallucinosis. A condition of more or less persistent hallucinations.

hallux. The great toe.

ham. 1. The back part of the thigh above the knee and below the buttock. 2. A vernacular term for the hip, thigh, or buttock.

hammertoe. A condition, usually of the second toe, in which the last two segments are bent down.

hamster. A short-tailed animal of the rodent family with large cheek pouches. It is native to Europe, Western Asia, and Africa. Because it is susceptible to a variety of germs, it is used for laboratory purposes.

harelip. A vertical gap or gaps in the lip resembling a rabbit's lip. —*acquired h.* Caused by an accident. —*congenital h.* Present at birth as the result of failure of fusion of the parts of the lip normally separated during development of the fetus. Often associated with cleft palate. May be of varying degrees from a small notch to an open gap extending to the nostril. —*double h.* Two gaps, one on each side of the lip.

hay fever. An acute involvement of the eyes, nose, and throat, an allergy to pollen. Generally, there are three types: —*fall h.f.* Occurring between the middle of August and the first of October and caused by ragweed pollen. —*summer* *h.f.* Starting in the middle of May and lasting to the middle of July, and caused by grass pollen, also called *rose fever*. —*spring h.f.* Starting in March and ending in May, and caused by tree pollen. The symptoms are sneezing, running, or clogging of the nose, itching and tearing of the eyes, mild cough. Also called *allergic rhinitis*.

head. 1. The uppermost part of the body that contains the brain, the organs of hearing, smell, sight, taste, and part of the organs of speech. 2. The top, beginning, or the most obvious or prominent part of anything.

headache. Pain in the head. Also called *cephalalgia*. —*histamine h*. Characterized by sudden onset of pain in the temple, neck, face, and one eye; tearing and congestion of that eye; clogged nostril; and swelling of the temple veins. Thought to follow the release of histamine into the bloodstream. —*ocular h*. Pain in head that results from disease or defects of the eyes. —*post traumatic h*. A continuous or recurring headache that often follows injury to the head. —*sick h*. Another name for migraine. It is also called *bilious headache, blind headache, migrainous headache*.

healing. The process of making whole or getting well; restoring to normal as in the closing of a wound, or the union of a broken bone. —*h. by first intention*. The union of wound edges that are held together by stitches or clips. This type of healing is feasible only when the skin edges are not too widely separated by the wound. —*h. by second intention*. The closure of a wound when the edges remain separated. This type of healing occurs after there is filling of the wound from its bottom by newly formed tissue to the level of the skin edges so that the skin can grow properly over the unhealed area.

heart. A hollow, muscular organ that pumps blood through the blood vessels, and is covered by a tough, loose sac of tissue, the *pericardium*. The heart consists of two halves each divided into a small chamber, the *atrium*, and a large chamber, the *ventricle*. There are therefore four chambers in all. The small chambers empty into the large chambers on each side, and the communication between the two is guarded by a valve. On the right side the valve is known as the *tricuspid*, and is composed of three small sections. On the left, the valve is called the *mitral*, and is composed of two small sections. The right atrium receives from the veins blood that has been depleted of oxygen. It forces the blood into the right ventricle from which it is expelled forcefully through the *pulmonary artery* into the lungs where new oxygen is picked up by the blood. The freshly oxygenated blood circulates back via the *pulmonary veins* into the left atrium and then into the left ventricle from which it is pumped into the aorta and thus through all of the arteries of the body and, depleted of oxygen, into the veins until it returns to the right atrium. —*h. disease.* There are two general types: that caused by forces at work outside of the heart, as compression, twisting of the heart, or high pressure of the blood; and that caused by disease within the heart, as of the heart muscle, valves, or arteries that supply the heart muscle with blood.

heart block. The beat of the heart depends primarily upon an electrical impulse that arises in the region of the atria and is transmitted to the ventricles. Normally, there is a pause in the passage of this impulse from one chamber to the other. In the first stage of heart block, this pause is prolonged; in the second, beats are actually dropped out; in the third, the atrium beats at a rhythm entirely independent of that of the ventricle. There are many types of heart block depending upon how complete the barrier is between the atrium and ventricle. Heart block may be due to disease within the heart muscle, to clots in the heart muscle blood vessels, or to injuries; and, at times, to a defect in the conduction system of the heart. The seriousness of heart block depends entirely upon its cause and degree. At all times, heart block interferes with the normal functioning of the body.

heartburn. A burning sensation beneath the breastbone, or over the middle chest on the left side usually related to muscular spasm of the gullet. Also called *gastric pyrosis*.

heart murmur. An abnormal sound heard through the stethoscope over the region of the heart. Murmurs are of many varieties and are ordinarily due to distortion in the valves of the heart.

heart rate. The number of heart beats per minute as detected by stethoscope over the region of the heart or by the fingertips at the wrist. Normal is 64-88.

heart sound. There are ordinarily two sounds heard on listening to the heart described as *lub-dub*. The first sound is long, and deep in pitch. It is thought to be caused by the contraction of the ventricle and the closure of the valve between ventricle and atrium. The second sound is shorter, and more highly pitched and has a snapping quality. It is thought to be caused by the closure of the valves between the left ventricle and the aorta after the blood has been forced into the aorta.

heat prostration. A condition resulting from exposure to high temperature that is characterized by a cold, clammy skin, a high temperature by rectum but a normal temperature by mouth, anxiety, and restlessness. Also called *heat exhaustion.*

hebephrenia (*hee-buh-free'nih-uh*). A type of schizophrenia that occurs in young people around the age of puberty, characterized by infantile behavior and thinking, silliness, smiling, undue laughing, untidiness, masturbation, hallucinations, secretiveness.

heliotherapy. The treatment of disease by exposing the body to sunlight, used in certain forms of tuberculosis.

helminthiasis (*hehl-mihn-thigh'uh-sihss*). The condition caused by the presence of parasitic worms in the body.

helminthology. The study of parasitic worms.

helotomy (*hee-laht'uh-mih*). The surgical cutting of a corn.

hemangiectasis (*hee-maan jih-ehk'tuh-sihss*). The excessive widening or enlargement of blood vessels, as the widened veins about the nose of a drinker.

hemangioma (*hee-maan-jih-oh'muh*). A tumor composed of blood vessels, as the *strawberry mole.*

hemarthrosis (*hee-mahr-throh'sihss*). The accumulation of blood in a joint.

hematemesis (*heh-muh-tehm'eh-sihss*). The vomiting of blood.

hematic. Having the color of, full of, or relating to blood.

hematinic. Any agent that tends to increase the hemoglobin content of blood.

hematocolpos (*hee-muh-tuh-kahl'puhs*). A collection of blood in the vagina.

hematocrit. The percentage of the total volume of blood composed of the blood cells after being separated from the serum in a centrifuge. The range is normally from 40 to 60 per cent. An important determination in the diagnosis of various blood diseases.

hematologist. A specialist in the study of blood and its diseases.

hematology. The study of blood, its functions, nature, and diseases.

hematoma (*hee-muh-toh'muh*). A tumor-like swelling that consists of blood that has flown out of a ruptured blood vessel. Usually caused by injury. Often appears at the site of a heavy blow.

hematuria (*hee-muh-too'rih-uh*). The presence of whole blood in the urine, frequently associated with kidney disease.

hemianesthesia (*hehm-ih-aan-uhss-thee'zhuh*). A loss of sensation in a longitudinal half of the body, caused by hysteria or injury to part of the brain.

hemianopsia (*hehm-ih-aa-nahp'sih-uh*). Blindness in half of each eye. May be the outer halves, the inner halves, the inner half of one and the outer half of the other.

hemicolectomy (*hehm-ih-koh-lehk'tuh-mih*). The surgical removal of half of the large intestine. Usually performed because of tumor growths.

hemicrania. Pain or headache on one side of the head only. Another name for *migraine*.

hemiglossectomy. Removal by surgery of one longitudinal half of the tongue.

hemiplegia (*hehm-ih-plee'jih-uh*). Paralysis of one side of the body. May be *spastic* from a birth injury, or occur later in life from an injury to various parts of the brain or the spinal cord.

hemisection. The dividing into two longitudinal halves.

hemithyroidectomy. The surgical removal of one of the two lobes of the thyroid gland.

hemochromatosis. A disease characterized by the deposit in the skin of one of the pigments of the blood causing a brownish discoloration. Often associated with diabetes. Also called *bronze diabetes*.

hemoglobin. A pigment contained within the red blood cells that has the vital property of combining with, and releasing, oxygen. It is this pigment that gives the red blood cell its color, and by virtue of which oxygen is taken from the air and given off to the cells in the body as needed. Chemically it is a combination of protein and iron salt.

hemoglobinemia. A condition in which the hemoglobin is dissolved out of the red blood cells and is suspended in the serum of the blood. This condition occurs in various forms of anemia and from other causes.

hemoglobinometer (*hee-muh-gloh-bih-nahm'ih-tuhr*). Any instrument used to determine the concentration of hemoglobin in the blood. The simplest of these is a piece of blotting paper with which a drop of blood is daubed. The color of the blot is compared with a color chart to reveal the concentration of hemoglobin. The lighter the color, the smaller is the percentage of hemoglobin indicated. There are many other more accurate methods, most of which employ a color scale.

hemoglobinuria (*hee-muh-gloh-bih-nyou'rih-uh*). The presence of hemoglobin in the urine due either to the destruction of red cells or to the solution of hemoglobin out of the red cells. —*epidemic h.* Occurring in the newborn, associated with blueness of the skin, nervous symptoms, jaundice. Also called *Winckles disease.* —*march h.* Occurring in attacks noted especially in soldiers after prolonged marching. —*nocturnal h.* A form occurring in attacks at night. —*paroxysmal h.* A type that recurs in attacks following exposure to cold or undue exertion. Often caused by a late stage of syphilis. —*toxic h.* Due to various types of poisoning.

hemolysis (*hee-mahl'ih-sihss*). The destruction of red blood cells with the escape of hemoglobin.

hemolyze (*hee'muh-lighz*). To produce hemolysis.

hemopericardium. Blood in the heart sac.

hemoperitoneum (*hee-muh-pehr-ih-tuh-nee'uhm*). A collection of blood in the abdominal cavity.

hemophilia (*hee-muh-fihl'ih-uh*). An inherited disease occurring only in males, transmitted from generation to generation by females. It is characterized by a prolonged bleeding-time and an unusually long delay in the time taken for the blood to clot. The disease with which the Spanish royal family was plagued for many generations. Also called the *bleeding disease.*

hemoptysis (*hih-mahp'tih-sihss*). The spitting up of blood, usually from the voice box, windpipe, breathing tubes, or lungs. Occurs in tuberculosis, cancer, some stages of pneumonia, and disease of the above-mentioned organs.

hemorrhage (*hehm'awr-rihdj*). Bleeding. An escape of blood from blood vessels.

hemorrhoidectomy (*hehm-uh-roy-dehk'tuh-mih*). The surgical removal of piles.

hemorrhoids (*hehm'uh-royds*). A varicose vein condition (enlargement and excessive widening of the veins) of the lower part of the rectum and the anus. Commonly called *piles.* —*external h.* Those situated below the muscle of the anus. —*internal h*. Those situated above the muscle of the anus.

hemostat (*hee'muh-staat*). An agent or instrument that stops the flow of blood, as the styptic pencil commonly used to stop bleeding in shaving; in surgery, a clamp, forceps.

hemothorax (*hee-muh-thaw'raaks*). An accumulation of blood in the space between the lungs and the chest wall.

heparin (*hehp'uh-rihn*). A substance normally present in the liver and other tissues whose function is to prevent the clotting of blood, i.e., to help maintain the blood liquid within the blood vessels. Heparin is isolated as a drug and used in those conditions where there is a tendency for blood clots to form and also in blood transfusions to prevent the clotting of blood.

hepatitis (*hehp-uh-tigh'tihss*). Inflammation of the liver. —*amebic h*. A widespread inflammation of the liver due to a disease-producing ameba, *Endameba histolytica*. If the condition is not cleared, abscesses may form in the liver. —*epidemic h*. An epidemic disease, probably caused by a virus, occurring with chills, fever, a variety of stomach and intestinal symptoms and, most often, jaundice. Also called *infectious jaundice*.

hepatoma (*hehp-uh-toh'muh*). Any tumor that has its origin in the liver. May vary from a simple, unimportant enlargement to a dangerous cancer.

hepatomegaly (*hehp-uh-toh-mehg'uh-lih*). Enlargement of the liver. Occurs in certain diseases of the liver itself, heart disease, blood diseases, and various infections.

hermaphrodite. An individual showing both ovary and testis tissues. Common in lower forms of animal life. In human beings the more frequent occurrence is the *pseudohermaphrodite*, the individual who has external genitals of one sex and internal sex glands of the other.

hernia. The abnormal protrusion of a part or an organ through the wall of the cavity in which it is contained and beyond its normal confines. Also called *rupture*. Commonest variety is the *inguinal hernia* in which the intestine pushes through a defect in the low abdominal wall and protrudes as a mass in the groin.

hernioplasty. An operation for the repair of a rupture.

herpes (*huhr'peez*). An inflammation of the skin or the lining tissues characterized by groups of small blisters. There are many types of herpes, and the commonest are *h. simplex*, seen particularly around the lips, often following a cold or intestinal upset, probably due to a virus, ordinarily called a *cold sore*; *h. zoster*, a condition in which the blisters follow the course of a nerve as often seen in the region of the ribs, are accompanied by severe pain, and are usually the result of a virus infection. Commonly called *shingles*.

heterometropia (*heht-uh-ruh-mih-troh'pih-uh*). A condition in which each eye requires a different lens prescription.

heterophoria (*heht-uh-ruh-faw'rih-uh*). A condition in which there is an imbalance of the muscles of the eye resulting in a tendency of the eye to turn away from the position that is correct for binocular vision. Noticeable only when one eye is covered, at which time, the uncovered eye will turn to one side or the other, up or down.

heterosexuality. Sexual desire for one of the opposite sex. "Normal" desire of man for woman, woman for man.

hiccup, hiccough. A sudden pulling down of the diaphragm that occurs in spasms, causing air to be sucked into the lungs in gulps, followed by a quick closure of the windpipe.

hidrosis. 1. The production and excretion of sweat. 2. An unusual amount of sweating.

hip. 1. The upper part of the thigh where it unites with the buttock. 2. The hip-joint.

Hirschsprung's disease. *See* DILATATION.

hirsuties (*huhr-soo'shih-eez*). An excessive growth of hair. Also called *hypertrichosis*.

histologist. A specialist in histology.

histology. The science that deals with the microscopic structure of tissues.

history. The story obtained from a patient concerning his health now and in the past, and the symptoms of his disease.

hives. A condition of the skin manifested by small and large, white, raised areas surrounded by zones of blushing-red that are very itchy. These may occur singly, in crops, on one part of the body, or all over the body. Due to allergy. Also called *urticaria*.

homosexuality. The state of being in love with or sexually attracted to members of one's own sex.

hookworm. *See* NECATORIASIS.

hordeolum (*hawr-dee'uh-luhm*). A sty. A tiny boil of the lid near a lash.

hormone. A chemical product of an organ or of special cells, as glands, excreted directly into the blood stream and carried by the blood stream for a specific effect on cells remote from its origin. Each hormone has a specific, single function. There are many hormones produced in the body, the most common of which are the thyroid hormone, the pituitary hormone, and the hormones produced by the ovaries and the testes.

house physician. A doctor who lives in the hospital and is available at all times as an intern.

humerus (*hyou'muh-ruhss*). The arm bone.

humpback, hunchback. *See* KYPHOSIS.

hydatid. A cyst that is formed in tissues due to infestation by a tapeworm transmitted to man from dog. It contains a watery liquid and a number of small hook-shaped structures that are parts of the developing worm. May occur in many organs, such as the lungs and the liver.

hydragogue. A strong laxative that causes the discharge of large amounts of fluid, as Epsom salts.

hydrargyria (*high-drahr-jigh'rih-uh*). Long-standing poisoning with mercury.

hydrarthrosis. An accumulation of fluid in a joint, as "water on the knee."

hydrocele (*high'druh-seel*). An accumulation of fluid in the sac that surrounds the testes within the scrotum.

hydrocephaly (*high-druh-sehf'ah-lih*). An accumulation beyond normal of the fluid that circulates within the brain and the spinal canal, causing increased pressure within the brain. Blockage of the normal exits for this fluid results in its accumulation. A defect of the exits may occur in the newborn, producing an unusually large head. If the pressure is not relieved after a certain point, death ensues.

hydrodipsomania. Attacks of uncontrollable thirst seen often in epilepsy and schizophrenia.

hydrophobia. 1. A morbid fear of water. 2. A virus disease transmitted to man by the bite of infected dogs. Also called *rabies*.

hydrotherapy. The treatment of disease by means of water, as the whirlpool bath, alternating hot and cold needle showers. Used especially in returning muscles and joints to normal activity after injury or disease and in the mentally disturbed.

hydrothorax. A collection of watery fluid in the space between the lungs and chest wall.

hymen. A thin tissue partition that blocks the opening of the vagina. Usually this has a small opening of its own that may be of several forms: circular, crescent, oval, zigzag. The opening in the hymen may be single or multiple; there may be no opening, in which case the hymen is *imperforate*.

hymenectomy (*high-muh-nehk'tuh-mih*). The surgical removal of the hymen.

hymenotomy. The surgical opening of the hymen.

hyoid (*high'oyd*). A bone between the root of the tongue and the voice box that helps to support the tongue and is an anchorage for some of the muscles of the tongue.

hypacusia (*hihp-uh-kyou'zih-uh*). Impairment of hearing.

hypalgesia (*hihp-aal-jee'zih-uh*). A reduced sensitivity to pain.

hyperacidity. An increased amount of acid, as "acid stomach."

hyperacuity (*high-puhr-uh-kyou'uh-tih*). Unusual sharpness of vision.

hyperacusia (*high-puhr-uh-kyou'zih-uh*). Unusual acuteness of hearing.

hyperemesis (*high-puhr-ehm'eh-sihss*). Undue amount of vomiting. —*h. gravidarum.* Pernicious vomiting of pregnancy.

hyperemia (*high-puhr-ee'mih-uh*). An oversupply of blood to a part with an increase in size of the blood vessels. This may be normal, as in blushing, and is called *active h.,* or it may be abnormal, as in heart failure or other conditions where the veins are blocked so that the blood backs up into the arteries, and is called *passive h.*

hyperglycemia (*high-puhr-gligh-see'mih-uh*). Excess sugar in the blood, as in *diabetes mellitus. See also* DIABETES.

hyperhidrosis (*high-puhr-hih-droh'sihss*). Excessive sweating. The sweat often accumulates as visible drops upon the skin.

hyperinsulinism (*high-puhr-ihn'syou-lihn-ihsm*). A condition manifest in attacks of loss of consciousness that may be accompanied by convulsions. Hyperinsulinism results from excess production of insulin and is treated with large amounts of sugar.

hyperkeratosis (*high-puhr-kehr-uh-toh'sihss*). 1. Overgrowth and enlargement of the transparent part of the eye. 2. Overgrowth of the upper, horny layer of the skin, as warts.

hypermastia. 1. Unusually large breasts. 2. The presence of more than two breasts.

hypermetropia. Farsightedness, due to an eyeball whose back-to-front diameter is abnormally short. Because of this condition the image falls behind the retina rather than upon it, as is normal. In order to correct hypermetropia, it is necessary to use a convex lens (as the ordinary magnifying glass) that brings the image from behind the retina directly upon it.

hypermotility. Increased movement, as increased activity of the intestine or stomach.

hypernephroma (*high-puhr-nehf-roh'muh*). A tumor of the kidney or other organs in which the cells resemble the cells of the adrenal gland. May be very serious.

hyperperistalsis (*high-puhr-pehr-uh-staal'sihss*). The intestinal tract and stomach have a normal rhythmic motion that serves to push their contents on and also to reduce them to a finer grade. This process is called *peristalsis*. When the rate and depth of this movement is greater than normal, the condition is called *hyperperistalsis*.

hyperpiesia (*high-puhr-pigh-ee'zhuh*). A state of unusually high blood pressure.

hyperpituitarism (*high-puhr-pih-too'ih-tuh-rihsm*). A condition in which certain cells of the pituitary gland are overactive. May result in a number of abnormal conditions, such as *gigantism* and *acromegaly*.

hyperplasia (*high-puhr-play'zhih-uh*). An increase in the size of a tissue or organ due to an increase in the number of cells, in contrast to an increase in size due to an increase in the size of the cells or of the units of a tissue or organ, a condition called *hypertrophy*

hyperpnea (*high-puhr-pnee'uh*). Hard breathing characterized by an increase in the depth of the inhalation.

hypersensitivity. The state of being unusually sensitive; most commonly means allergy.

hypersthenia. A condition of unusual strength or tone of the body. Seen among professional acrobats and strong men.

hypertension. High blood pressure.

hyperthyroidism. An abnormal condition of excessive activity of the thyroid gland.

hypertrichosis (*high-puhr-trigh-koh'sihss*). Excessive hairiness.

hypertrophy (*high-puhr'troh-fih*). An increase in size of an organ due to enlargement of its constituent cells. The muscles of an athlete exhibit hypertrophy.

hypesthesia (*hihp-uhs-thee'zhuh*). A decrease in the capacity for physical sensation.

hypnagogic (*hihp-nuh-gahdj'ihk*). Inducing sleep, as a situation or medication.

hypnosis. A trance or a state of sleep that is brought about in an individual by the hypnotist through verbal suggestion or by the person's concentration upon an object. It is characterized by ready response to suggestions made by the hypnotist.

hypochondriasis (*high-puh-kahn-drigh'uh-sihss*). A condition in which the patient is overconcerned with his own health and believes himself to be afflicted with some grave disease. Caused by an underlying psychological derangement.

hypochondrium (*high-puh-kahn'drih-uhm*). An area of the abdomen just below the ribs limited to the outer two-thirds of the abdominal wall.

hypodermic. 1. Relating to the area beneath the skin. 2. Introduced under the skin. 3. Injection under the skin. 4. The syringe used for injection under the skin, colloquially abbreviated to "hypo."

hypogastrium. An area of the abdomen below the navel and above the pubis.

hypoglossal. Situated under the tongue.

hypoglycemia (*high-puh-gligh-see'mih-uh*). A condition characterized by subnormal sugar content of the blood due either to excess use of sugar by the body or to an interference with the formation of sugar in the liver. The normal fasting sugar content of the blood is between 80 and 120 milligrams per cent. Hypoglycemia appears when the sugar level drops to 60 or lower. The symptoms are dizziness, alternating flushing and pallor of the face, nervousness, excessive sweating, hunger, and, at times, loss of consciousness. The treatment for the immediate attack is sugar by mouth and/or vein.

hypomastia (*high-puh-maas'tih-uh*). Unusual smallness of the breast.

hypophysis (*high-pahf'ih-sihss*). The pituitary gland.

hypopituitarism (*hih-poh-pih-too'ih-tuh-rihsm*). A condition in which a part of the pituitary gland does not produce enough hormone. Some of the common symptoms are impotence, sterility, absence of the menstrual cycle, hypoglycemia, and a general tendency of the tissues and the organs to shrink.

hypoplasia (*high-puh-play'zhih-uh*). The failure of tissue to develop completely. For example, a hypoplastic womb is one that has failed to develop to normal size and resembles that of an infant.

hyposensitization. A process used in treatment of allergic conditions in which small amounts of the material to which a patient is allergic are given in gradually increasing doses at regular intervals until his allergy to the material is greatly reduced, as in the injection treatment for hay fever.

hypospadias (*high-poh-spay'dih-uhs*). An abnormality of the penis existing from birth in which its passageway opens on the lower surface of the penis rather than on its tip. Also a malformation in which the passageway from the bladder in a female opens into the vagina.

hypotension. An abnormally low blood pressure.

hypothyroidism. A condition resulting from deficient production of thyroid hormone, causing a low metabolism, sluggishness, mental dullness, weight gain, sexual deficiency, brittleness, and tendency to loss of hair. Treated with thyroid extract.

hysterectomy (*hihss-tuhr-ehk'tuh-mih*). A total or partial surgical removal of the womb, performed through an incision in the abdominal wall or through the vagina.

hysteria. A condition, the result of deep emotional conflict, characterized by extreme emotionalism and often disturbances of the muscle system, as paralysis of various organs (stomach, intestine, heart, and others). There may also be disturbances of the various senses. Examples of the latter are hysterical blindness, deafness, and loss of sensation in various areas of the body.

hysterosalpingectomy (*hihss-tuh-ruh-saal-pihn-jehk'tuh-mih*). Surgical removal of the womb and tubes.

I

ichthyosis (*ihk-thih-oh'sihss*). An abnormality of the skin occurring at birth, characterized by dry, scaly, leathery skin, worsening in cold weather. Called *fish skin, alligator skin.*

iconolagny. Stimulation of sexual desire by the sight of statues or pictures.

icteric. Relating to or characterized by jaundice.

icterus. Jaundice, a yellow coloration of the skin, due to interference with the passage of bile from the gall bladder into the intestinal tract, excessive destruction of red blood cells, or injury to the liver.

id. The early, primitive mind consisting of a maze of instincts and only vaguely aware of reality. *See also* EGO.

idiocy. Mental deficiency in which the mental age is under three and the I.Q. under 25. Ordinarily appears at birth and is accompanied by physical defects. There are various types of idiocy, as Mongolian idiocy, hydrocephalic idiocy, and others. *See* INTELLIGENCE QUOTIENT.

idiogamist (*id-ih-ahg'uh-mihst*). A male who is capable of having sexual intercourse only with his wife or with a few women; he is impotent with women in general.

ileitis (*ihl-ih-igh'tihss*). Inflammation of the lower portion of the small intestine.

ileocolitis (*ihl-ih-oh-koh-ligh'tihss*). An inflammation of the lower part of the small intestine and the large intestine.

ileocolostomy (*ihl-ih-oh-koh-lahs'tuh-mih*). The surgical establishment of a communication between the lower part of the small intestine and the large intestine. This operation is performed in order to provide a shunt for the contents of the intestinal tract around a diseased area in the first part of the large intestine, or the lower part of the small intestine.

ileostomy. An incision through the abdominal wall into the lower part of the small intestine that is kept open as an artificial anus.

ileum (*ihl′ih-uhm*). The lower part of the small intestine.

ileus. A condition characterized by marked bloating, severe pain, continuous vomiting that becomes fecal, an increasing pulse rate, and severe sickness ending fatally unless relieved. Ileus is caused by obstruction of the intestine by tumor, adhesion, or serious infection. At times ileus results from paralysis of the bowel, an unfortunate side-effect of abdominal surgery.

ilium. 1. The flank. 2. The upper wide part of the hipbone that can easily be felt by pressing into the flank and down.

illusion. A false interpretation of a real sensation. Example: when one is on a motionless train next to another train just starting off, the sense that one is moving backward and the other train is standing still.

image, imago (*ih-may′goh*). The picture of a loved or hated person formed in infancy and preserved indefinitely in the individual's unconscious. Commonest imagos are those of parents or parent substitutes.

imbecility. A grade of mental deficiency in which the mental age is between three and seven years and the I.Q. between 25 and 49. This degree of deficiency stands between idiocy and moronity. *See* INTELLIGENCE QUOTIENT.

imbrication. A method of surgically closing wounds in which the tissues are sewed in overlapping layers, resembling the lamination of wood.

immobilization. The act of making immovable, as in the use of splints about a break in a bone.

immune. Protected against a disease; safe from attack.

immunity. The state of a living organism in which it resists and overcomes infection. There are two primary types of immunity. —*active i.* The state of protection arising either through infection or by a series of injections, as the immunity of an individual who has had diphtheria, or who has had the diphtheria injections. *—passive i.* The state of protection, usually a temporary one, derived by the injection of antibodies. Example, the immunity conferred by the injection of *tetanus antitoxin.* Tetanus antibodies (antitoxin), produced in the blood stream of the horse by injection of tetanus poison, are injected in the human as a serum. This, in effect, is a short-term loan of protection.

immunologist. A specialist in the science of immunity.

immunology. The science that embraces the study of the processes by which the body overcomes infection.

immunotransfusion. The transfusion with blood from an individual who has before been made immune by inoculation or infection with a given disease. Example, the transfusion with blood from an individual who has had scarlet fever as a protective device against scarlet fever, or as an aid in treating the condition.

imperforate. Where the normal opening does not exist, as "imperforate hymen."

impermeable. Not permitting passing through, commonly used in reference to a membrane or tissue.

impetigo (*ihm-puh-tigh′goh*). An inflammation of the skin characterized by blisters of varying shapes on various areas of the body. *—i. contagiosa.* A highly contagious form of impetigo in which there are small blisters whose contents turn to pus, ooze, and form crusts with a golden yellow color. Ordinarily found on exposed parts, as the face and hands. Usually heals without any aftereffects. *—i. herpetiformis.* A rare skin condition characterized by very tiny pus-filled blisters that tend to unite in circular groups. Most often found in pregnant women. Commonly fatal. *—i. neonatorum.* A form occurring in the newborn in which the blisters are of large size.

impotence. Incapacity for sexual intercourse in the man, most frequently psychological in origin.

inanition. An abnormal state of the body due to lack of food and/or water. Starvation is a form of inanition.

incarceration. The unusual imprisonment of a part, seen often in rupture where the loop of intestine is caught in a pouch of tissue, that does not permit it to move back to its normal position.

incipient. Beginning, about to appear, as incipient tuberculosis.

incontinence. The inability to control normal evacuation, as of the bowel or bladder.

incrustation. The formation of a hard coating or a crust on a wet, weeping wound; a scab.

incubation. That stage of an infectious disease which lasts from the time the germ finds its way into the body until the appearance of the first symptoms.

indication. Any aspect of a disease, such as a symptom or cause, that points out its treatment.

induration (*ihn-dyou-ray'shuhn*). The hardening of an area caused by inflammation or tumor growth, as the hard and painful area surrounding a boil.

inebriation. Drunkenness; intoxication.

infantile paralysis. See Poliomyelitis.

infantilism. The continuation of infantile or childish characteristics into adult life, marked by physical, mental, and sexual underdevelopment, and caused by a number of conditions, as thyroid deficiency, chronic infection, pituitary deficiency, and others. Also called *Lorain syndrome*.

infarct. A region of decaying tissue due to an interference with blood flow, as complete obstruction of the artery that supplies the blood to, or obstruction of the vein that drains the blood from, a part.

infarction. The process following the obstruction of a blood vessel that leads to the development of tissue destruction, the infarct.

infection. 1. The implantation of a germ. 2. The communication of a disease from one person to another. 3. The spread of disease from one area of the body to another.

infertility. Sterility; the inability to bear or produce progeny.

infiltration. A process by which substances pass into cells or into the spaces around cells. These substances may be normal but present in an unusual amount, or they may be foreign. Examples: the deposit of calcium in an area of infection such as in tuberculosis; the passage of urine from a ruptured bladder into tissue spaces where it does not normally occur.

inflammation. The reaction of tissue to injury, consisting of certain observable findings; heat at the area of injury, redness, swelling, and pain.

influenza. An epidemic disease characterized by inflammation of the lining tissue of the nose, throat, bronchial tubes, accompanied by cough, phlegm, discharge from the nose, fever, pain in the muscles, and prostration. At times the symptoms may be chiefly of the nervous system. Influenza is caused by a virus of various types called influenza A, B, C, and so on. Common complications are pneumonia, pleurisy, infection of the middle ear, and neuritis.

ingestion. The act of taking substances, especially food, into the body by mouth, as eating, taking a medicine by mouth, drinking.

inguinal (*ihn'gwih-nuhl*). Referring to the groin.

inhalant (*ihn-hay'luhnt*). 1. That which is inhaled, as a medicine or agent that may do injury. 2. Related to, or used for, inhaling.

inhibition. The thwarting of an instinctual impulse by the individual's unconscious mind. A means of preventing conflict between the ego and the id. *See also* EGO.

innervation. 1. The distribution of nerves to a part. 2. The amount of nervous stimulation received by a part.

innocuous. Harmless.

inoculation. The act of introducing a germ or other agent into the body, usually with the intention of producing a mild form of the disease as a means of immunity. Examples: typhoid injections, hay fever injections.

inoperable. A condition in which the outlook is unfavorable if an operation is performed.

insemination. The introduction of semen into the vagina; impregnation. —*artificial i.* The injection of semen into the vagina or womb by the use of an instrument to induce pregnancy.

inspissate. Thickening by the loss of fluid, as inspissated mucus in the bronchial tubes, hardening of mucus due to a loss of its fluid part.

instillation. Introducing a liquid into a cavity, drop by drop, as dropping medicine into an eye.

insufflation. The act of blowing a gas, powder, or vapor into a body cavity, as spraying a powdered medicine into the nose.

integument (*ihn-tehg′you-muhnt*). A covering, particularly the skin.

intelligence quotient. A figure used to indicate a person's intelligence, arrived at by dividing the mental age by the age in years. There are three grades of mental deficiency: idiocy, imbecility, and moronity. The I.Q. of these three fall below 69. Above 69 the classification is: dull normal, 70 to 90; normal, 90 to 110; superior, 110 to 125; very superior, 125 to 140; and genius, 140 and above.

intercurrent. Taking place between, as a disease occurring during the existence of another disease in the same person.

interdigitation (*ihn-tuhr-dihj-ih-tay′shuhn*). Dovetailing, as the fingers of one hand with those of the other.

intermenstrual. Between the menstrual periods.

intermittent. Taking place at intervals, as intermittent fever, intermittent insanity, intermittent depression.

internist. A physician who specializes in nonsurgical internal medicine.

intertrigo (*ihn-tuhr-trigh′goh*). A red eruption of the skin produced by the rubbing together of parts. Examples: intertrigo of the thighs, particularly in fat people; intertrigo under the breasts, where the breast rubs against the chest wall.

intestine. That part of the digestive tube that extends from the lower end of the stomach to the anus. The small intestine is 20 feet long and extends from the lower end of the stomach to the large intestine. The small intestine is divided into the *duodenum*, the *jejunum*, and the *ileum*. The large intestine is about five feet long and consists of the *cecum* from which hangs the *appendix*, the *colon*, and the *rectum*. The intestinal wall is composed of four coats, an inner mucous coat, a coat that contains most of the glands, a muscular coat, and an outer serous coat. Most of the digestive processes occur in the duodenum. Within the colon, final stages of breakdown of food occur with the aid of bacteria that normally live there.

intima (*ihn′tih-muh*). The inner one of the three coats of the wall of a blood vessel.

intoxication. 1. Poisoning, as by a serum, drug, or alcohol. 2. The acute condition produced by overindulgence in alcohol; drunkenness.

intracellular. Within a cell.

intrauterine (*ihn-truh-you′tuh-rihn*). Within the womb.

intravenous (*ihn-truh-vee′nuhss*). Within or into a vein, as an intravenous injection.

introitus (*ihn-troh′ih-tuhss*). An entrance, particularly the vaginal entrance.

intromission. The insertion of; the act of putting in; the introduction of one body into another.

introversion. Ordinarily, the instincts seek expression in the outer world of reality. When instinctual energy is re-routed toward the inner world of the individual, introversion has occurred. This results in a withdrawal of interest from the world about and a satisfaction with the inner world of phantasy. When extreme, it characterizes a number of psychoses, as schizophrenia.

intubation. The placement of a tube into a hollow organ to keep it open, especially the introduction of a tube into the windpipe to insure passage of air when an injury or disease threatens to close it, as in acute diphtheria or in severe allergic swelling.

intussusception (*ihn-tuhs-suh-sehp′shuhn*). Refers particularly to the slipping or passage of one part of the intestine into another. An illustration of intussusception is the partial closing of an extended pocket telescope. The symptoms of this condition are severe recurrent pain, vomiting, passage of blood and mucus through the rectum, and the presence of a sausage-shaped tumor in the lower abdomen. Usually occurs in infants and requires immediate surgery.

invagination (*ihn-vaaj-uh-nay'shuhn*). The act of becoming insheathed. *See* INTUSSUSCEPTION.

inversion. Used synonymously with sexual inversion. A routing of the sexual instinct toward persons in the image of one's self or of one's parent of the same sex. Homosexuality.

in vitro (*ihn-vee'troh*). A process or reaction that is carried out in the laboratory in a test tube.

in vivo (*ihn-vee'voh*). Within the living organism. Used in contrast to in vitro.

involution. 1. The change back to normal that certain organs undergo after fulfilling their function, as the womb after pregnancy, the breasts after breast-feeding is over. 2. The period or the process of decline and gradual decay that occurs generally in people after middle life.

iodism. A condition often resulting from prolonged use of iodine or its salts, characterized by excessive production of saliva, ache in the forehead, running nose, tearing eyes, occasionally a cough and a skin eruption.

ipsilateral. Situated on the same side, as symptoms that appear on the same side as the brain injury that causes them.

iridectomy (*ihr-ih-dehk'tuh-mih*). The surgical removal of a part of the colored portion of the eye, the *iris*.

iridocyclitis (*ihr-uh-doh-sigh-kligh'tihss*). Inflammation of the colored part of the eye and the muscle to which it is attached.

iridocystectomy (*ihr-uh-doh-sihss-tehk'tuh-mih*). An operation for making a new pupil.

iris. The colored, circular disc of the eye, suspended behind the transparent part of the eye, the *cornea*. Its hind surface rests on the lens of the eye and thus it separates the front chamber of the eye from the hind chamber. The iris consists of a mass of loose tissue and contains a set of circular muscles and a set of muscles that runs radially through it like the spokes of a wheel. These muscles control the size of the pupil.

iritis. An inflammation of the iris.

iritoectomy (*ihr-uh-toh-ehk'tuh-mih*). The removal of a part of the iris in cases where the pupil is closed over.

iron lung. A popular term for *respirator*, used to cause breathing in a patient whose muscles of breathing are paralyzed, by enclosing the patient's body up to the neck and, through changes in air pressure, forcing the chest to expand and contract. *See also* RESPIRATION.

ischium (*ihss'kih-uhm*). The bone upon which the body rests in sitting.

isotope (*igh'soh-tohp*). Any of the two or more forms of an element, having the same atomic number but a different atomic weight.

isthmus (*ihss'muhss*). The neck or the narrowed part of an organ, as the isthmus of the thyroid gland; a narrow, horizontal part of the gland connecting the two large sections of the gland similar to the crossbar of an H.

itch. An irritating sensation in the skin relieved by scratching.

J

jaundice. Yellowness of the skin, lining tissues, and secretions due to bile pigments in the blood. Generally jaundice has three essential causes: 1. Obstruction of bile flow into the intestinal tract with a damming back of the bile and eventually its appearance in the blood. 2. Unusual destruction of red blood cells with release into the blood of the cell-pigment that under normal circumstances is eventually transformed into bile. 3. Disease or injury to the liver cells that prevents them from manufacturing bile and therefore causes a damming back into the blood stream of the pigments ordinarily so used.

jaw. Applied to one of two bones that form the skeleton of the mouth: the *maxilla*, the upper jaw, and the *mandible*, the lower jaw.

jejunitis (*jee-joo-nigh'tihss*). Inflammation of the jejunum, the middle section of the small intestine.

jejunum (*jih-joo'nuhm*). The second division of the small intestine that extends between the duodenum and the ileum and is about 8 feet in length.

jockey strap. A suspensory. The name ordinarily given to a scrotum support.

joint. Ordinarily refers to an area of meeting of two different bones, structured for their easy movement upon one another. There are other immovable joints, as the lines of union between the various bones of the skull. Joints are of many types depending upon the type of motion they permit, as ball and socket joint, the arm with the shoulder; hinge joint, the knee.

joint mouse. A small body, free within a joint, ordinarily derived from the lining tissue within the joint. At times the joint mouse is hardened by calcification, producing pain and disturbance in the movement of the joint, and may require operation.

jugular (*joo'gyuh-luhr*). Relating to the throat, as the jugular vein.

juice. Usually refers to any of the secretions of the body, as stomach juice, intestinal juice, juice of the pancreas.

June cold. Another name for *rose fever*, a type of hay fever resulting from allergy to grass pollen. Appears in mid-May and ends in mid-July.

jungle rot. A term used by the military to denote a tropical fungus infection.

justa-major. Larger in every respect than normal. Applied to the bony pelvis.

justa-minor. Unusually small in all dimensions. Applied to the bony pelvis.

juxtaposition. State of being placed side by side, close together.

K

kala azar (*kah'lah ah-zahr'*). A tropical disease caused by a germ, *leishmania*. There are two types of this disease that affect the internal organs. One attacks children and adults in the Near East and the other attacks infants in Mediterranean countries. Generally, it is a serious and often fatal condition, with irregular fever, thinning of the blood, severe weight loss, and enlargement of the spleen and liver.

kaolin. A refined, powdered aluminum silicate used as a dusting powder for ulcerations and wounds that discharge freely, or internally as a soothing agent for inflammation of the intestines.

karaya gum (*kah-righ'uh*). A substance obtained from the sap of certain trees, having the property of absorbing large amounts of water. It is sometimes used as a laxative. Cosmetically, it is often used in hair preparations and is not infrequently the source of allergic conditions.

keloid (*kee'loyd*). A tumorous growth consisting of tough, scar tissue almost always occurring in the site of a scar. A keloid is raised, white or pink, and firm to the feel. It seems to occur most frequently on the upper part of the trunk and face, especially in Negroes, females, or young adults. Although unsightly, it in no way threatens life.

keratectomy. The surgical removal of part of the cornea, the transparent part of the eye.

keratinization (*kehr-uh-tihn-ih-zay'shuhn*). The development of a horny quality in tissues, as in the formation of warts or callouses.

keratitis. Inflammation of the cornea. This condition is due to infections, allergy, lack of vitamins, and injury.

keratoconjunctivitis. Inflammation of the transparent part of the eye, the lining tissue of the whites of the eye, and the underparts of the lids. A type called *epidemic k.* is caused by a virus that usually affects adults and runs a relatively short course.

keratoiritis (*kehr-uh-toh-igh-righ'tihss*). Combined inflammation of the cornea and the iris.

keratolytic. Any agent that causes the skin to shed, as the various ointments and liquids containing salicylic acid used as corn remedies.

keratome. A knife that has a blade resembling a mason's trowel used for cutting into the cornea during the operation for removing part of the iris.

keratoscleritis. An inflammation of the cornea and the white of the eye.

keratosis. Any disease of the skin that produces an overgrowth of a horny material as multiple warts, or painful thickening and cracking of the skin. In some of these conditions, especially those appearing in older people, a form of skin cancer may develop.

ketosis (*kih-toh'sihss*). Normally in the processes that the body employs to break down fats, substances called ketones result. Under ordinary circumstances these ketones are further broken down into innocuous carbon dioxide and water. Under certain circumstances, particularly in diabetes, this latter step is incomplete. As a result, there is a marked increase in ketones in the body and the condition *ketosis* sets in. If not cared for immediately, death may result.

ketosteroid (*kih-toh'stuh-royd*). The name of a large group of chemical substances produced by the body of primary importance to normal development, body functioning, and life. Among the ketosteroids are the hormones commonly used in the treatment of change of life in women; testosterone; and the newer hormones, such as cortisone.

kidney. One of a pair of organs situated in the back of the abdominal cavity, on either side of the spine, just below the spleen on the left and the liver on the right. The kidney is bean-shaped and weighs about a third of a pound. It is covered by a thick, tough, fibrous coat and is imbedded in fat. Its function is to help regulate the concentration of various constituents of the blood by excreting water and other products considered waste. It probably also furnishes substances that control the blood pressure. The unit of the kidney is known as the *renal corpuscle*, consisting of a *glomerulus* that is a tuft of capillary loop fitting like a fist into a palm, or *capsule*. This capsule is the end of a hollow tube through which passes the fluid from the blood contained in the glomerulus. Through a complicated system of merging with other such tubes the large collecting portion of the kidney, the *pelvis*, is attained. From the pelvis the fluid is led down a tube known as the *ureter* that empties into the bladder.

kinesthesia (*kihn-uhs-thee′zhuh*). The muscle sense. The sense of movement of muscle, recognition of weight, position, and resistance. Weight judging, or judging just how much to use the muscle to carry the arm to a certain point are examples of kinesthesia.

kiotomy (*kigh-aht′uh-mih*). The surgical removal of the uvula, the small tongue of tissue that hangs down from the soft palate at the back of the mouth.

kleptomania. Obsessive stealing. A morbid need to steal. A psychological disorder in which the things stolen usually have a symbolic value only since they are ordinarily useless or unimportant items.

kraurosis (*kraw-roh′sihss*). A hardening and shriveling process of the skin, usually due to a wasting away of glands. Frequently attacks the genitals of elderly women. Symptoms are itching, shriveling, and drying of the genitalia. Complete closure of the vagina may occur.

kyphosis. A curvature of the spine with the hump of the curve behind, usually in the upper part of the spine, in the region of the chest. Often the result of certain types of arthritis, tuberculosis, or bad posture. Also called *humpback, hunchback*.

L

labium. A lip, as the lips of the mouth. —*l. majus*. A fold of skin on either side of the vaginal opening arising just below the pubis. —*l. minus*. A fold of skin on either side of the vaginal opening arising on the inner surface of the *l. majus*.

labor. Childbirth. —*artificial l*. Childbirth aided by other than natural processes. —*dry l*. Childbirth in which there is an absence or deficiency in the normal amount of fluid, or in which there has been an early rupture of the bag of waters. —*l. pains*. The pains produced by the spasm of the womb during labor. —*precipitate l*. A sudden, rapid expulsion of the fetus.

labyrinth. 1. A maze; a complicated system of passageways connected with one another. 2. Such a system makes up part of the inner ear.

laceration. 1. A tear. 2. The act of tearing, as an injury that results in rupture of skin and muscle. —*l. of perineum*. The tearing through of the wall that separates the vagina from the rectum, often occurring during childbirth.

lacrimal. 1. (*adj.*) Relating to the tears or to the parts that secrete and convey the tears. 2. (*n.*) A bone on the side of the nose that makes up part of the eye socket.

lacrimation. Excessive flowing of tears.

lactation. 1. The production and secretion of milk. 2. The period of breast feeding; suckling.

lacteal (*lack'teel*). 1. Relating to milk. 2. One of numerous small ducts within the small intestine that take up and convey emulsified fat.

lactic acid. An acid normal to the blood and related to muscle fatigue. The acid is a colorless, almost odorless liquid, very thick, that mixes easily with water, and is used in contraceptive jellies to kill sperm, as an antiseptic for infected wounds, and as an addition to milk to make the curd smaller for infant-feeding.

lactobacillus. The name of a large family of germs capable of making lactic acid from starches and starchlike compounds. —*l. acidophilus.* A type of lactobacillus that curdles milk and that is used in the production of acidophilus milk. Some believe that it makes the secretion of the vagina acid and thus helps defend it against infection.

lactose. Milk sugar; a type of sugar found in milk used in infant-feeding formulas and often as a filler in pills and capsules.

lacuna. A small space or pit.

lagrippe (*lah-grihp'*). Influenza.

lameness. A weakness or partial disability of the leg so that the gait is no longer normal. Limping. May be due to shrinking of muscle, acute pain, disease, or any disturbance of the leg. Examples: lameness following a break of the leg bone, or the "falling asleep" of the leg.

laminectomy (*laam-uh-nehk'tuh-mih*). An operation in which the arches of the vertebrae are removed, often performed for the condition of slipped disc, and in preparation for fusion of the spine.

lancet. A puncturing knife, short and double-edged. A miniature type is used in puncturing the finger to obtain a small amount of blood for a blood count.

lanolin. The fat obtained from sheep's wool, commonly employed as the base of ointments and cosmetics.

lanugo (*luh-noo′goh*). A very fine growth of hair that covers the infant from its fifth month within the womb until shortly after birth.

laparotomy (*laap-uh-raht′uh-mih*). The surgical cutting into the abdominal cavity, either through the belly wall or flank. The initial stage of an operation on any organ or part within the abdominal cavity, as the removal of the gall bladder or stomach, or operations upon the intestines.

larva. The immature young of many animals, especially insects, that undergo a series of changes before reaching the adult stage. Maggots are larvae of flies; caterpillars of butterflies.

larvicide. Any agent or chemical that destroys the larvae of insects, such as demothing agents.

laryngectomy (*laar-ihn-jehk′tuh-mih*). The surgical removal of part or all of the voice box.

laryngismus (*laar-ihn-jihz′muhss*). A muscular spasm of the voice box. *l. stridulus.* A condition of the voice box characterized by periods of spasm and seen mostly in young children and infants with rickets. The symptoms are dramatic; a sudden crowing, deep breath followed by stoppage of breathing for several seconds; blueness of the skin followed by loud, long whistling breaths.

laryngitis (*laar-ihn-jigh′tihss*). Inflammation of the voice box caused by many conditions, as infection, allergy, injury, irritation.

laryngology (*laar-ihn-gahl′uh-jih*). The study of the structure, function, and diseases of the voice box.

laryngoscope (*luh-rihn′guh-skohp*). An instrument for examining the inside of the voice box composed of a mirror attached at an angle to a long handle.

laryngotomy (*laar-ihn-gaht′uh-mih*). An operation consisting of cutting into the larynx.

larynx. The voice box or organ that makes the voice possible;

specifically, the upper continuation of the windpipe extending to the root of the tongue, consisting of a number of pieces of gristle lined by a moist mucous tissue, that are moved by the muscles of the larynx. Within the voice box, the lining mucous membrane is thrown into folds that cross it from a common point in front, forming a "V" when seen from above. By virtue of the muscles these vocal cords can be brought close together or separated, producing changes in pitch. The space between the vocal cords is called the *rima glottidis*.

lateral. Relating, or belonging to, the side. Situated on a side. Example: Ears and arms are lateral organs; the eyes are lateral to the nose; the flank is lateral to the navel.

laudanum. A tincture of opium (10 to 20 per cent of opium in an alcoholic solution).

lavage (*lah-vahj'*). The washing out of an organ as the bowel, bladder, stomach, sinuses.

laxative. A mild cathartic; an agent that makes the bowels loose.

lead poisoning. A form of poisoning that may be *acute* and characterized by burning in the throat and metallic taste in the mouth followed by severe belly pain and perhaps collapse; or *chronic* when occurring in people who are exposed to small amounts of lead over a long period of time, as painters or miners. The symptoms appear gradually as dyspepsia, loss of appetite, weakness, and severe constipation accompanied by marked pain. Often a blue line appears in the gums; and various nervous symptoms may come on, as paralysis of the wrist or ankle, which causes the hand or foot to hang limp.

leg. The lower extremity; the part from the knee to the ankle.

leiomyoma (*ligh-oh-migh-oh'muh*). A tumor, not ordinarily dangerous to life, consisting largely of muscle cells that constitute the muscles not under the control of the will. Leiomyoma may be found wherever such muscle normally occurs, as the womb, intestine, stomach, bladder, under the skin, and at the hair follicles.

leiomyosarcoma (*ligh-oh-migh-oh-sahr-koh'muh*). A cancerous tumor made up of involuntary muscle cells, many of which are very immature. This immaturity makes the tumor dangerous since the cells may, and often do, grow wild.

Leishmania (*leesh-may'nih-uh*). A microscopic single-celled animal with a whiplike tail that propels it, producing disease in man. The malady is transmitted to man by the bite of a type of sand fly and is mostly confined to the tropics and semi-tropics.

lens. 1. A crystal or piece of glass that bends rays of light passing through it, as a magnifying glass, a reducing glass, or the glass used in spectacles. 2. The transparent egg-shaped body lying behind the pupil of the eye, called the *crystalline lens* of the eye. —*biconcave l.* A thick-edged lens having cupped surfaces, the bulge of the cups toward the interior of the lens resembling parentheses back to back, as)(. Called a *negative or minus lens*. This lens tends to lengthen the rays of light that pass through it, bending them upward. For this reason a biconcave lens is used to correct nearsightedness when the image passing through the lens of the eye falls *in front* of the retina. By use of a biconcave lens the image is made to fall farther back in the eye *upon* the retina. —*biconvex l.* The opposite of the biconcave, its cupped surfaces bulging outward as in a magnifying glass, as (). This lens has the property of bending light down and is used therefore in the correction of farsightedness where the image falls *behind* the retina. This lens will draw the image closer to the interior of the eye and make it fall *upon* the retina.

lenticular. 1. Resembling or relating to a lens. 2. Relating to the crystalline lens of the eye.

lentigo (*lehn-tigh'goh*). A freckle; a small patch of pigment occurring mainly on the face and hands.

leprosy. A disease mostly of tropical and subtropical countries. Infectious, caused by a specific germ, *Myobacterium* *leprae*, and characterized by affection of the skin and nerves. Also called *Hansen's disease*. —*lepromatous l.* A variety involving the skin in small tumor masses that break down and become ulcerations. Highly infectious. —*neural l.* The type of leprosy that involves the nerves, mostly causing loss of sensation and loss of nutrition to the skin with eventual deformities and falling off of parts, as the fingers, nose. Mildly or not infectious.

lesbianism. Homosexuality between women; unnatural affection between one woman and another. Also called *sapphism*, *tribadism*.

lesion. Any change in a tissue due to disease or injury, as a bullet wound, ulcer, cataract.

lethargy. An unusual state of stupor or drowsiness.

leukemia (*loo-kee'mih-uh*). A disease of blood-forming organs that results in an excessive production of white blood cells. Although normally a few undeveloped white blood cells are found in the blood, in leukemia their number is often large. Ordinarily, such immature white blood cells are present only in those organs that form white blood cells and are not discharged into the blood stream until they develop to maturity. There are a number of varieties of leukemia, but two types are common. —*lymphatic l.* A form in which the spleen and the lymph nodes are enlarged, and white blood cells without granules in their protoplasm, the *lymphocytes*, are increased in number. —*myelogenous l.* A form in which the white blood cells manufactured in the bone marrow are primarily involved, and many undeveloped white blood cells with granules in their protoplasm are present in the blood in great numbers. Both of these conditions are serious and eventually fatal.

leukoblast. A general term for the white blood cell that has not yet grown to maturity.

leukocyte. A general name for the white blood cells in the blood stream. These are divided into *nongranular leukocytes*, white blood cells that have no granules in their protoplasm, the *lymphocyte*, and the *monocyte; granular leukocytes*, white blood cells containing granules in their protoplasm, that may be *neutrophilic* where the granules stain with a neutral dye, *eosinophilic* where the granules stain red with an acid dye, and *basophilic* where the granules stain blue with an alkaline dye.

leukocytolysis (*loo-koh-sigh-tahl'ih-sihss*). The destruction of white blood cells.

leukocytosis (*loo-koh-sigh-toh'sihss*). An increase beyond normal in the number of white blood cells in the blood, characteristic of many infections and other ailments. Normal after meals and during pregnancy.

leukopenia (*loo-koh-pee'nih-uh*). A subnormal number of white blood cells in the blood. Occurs as a late stage of leukemia, certain types of allergy, and as a threatening condition in itself.

libido (*lih-bee'doh*). The energy of the sexual instincts (Freud), or psychic energy in general (Bleuler, Jung).

lichenification (*ligh-kuhn-ih-fih-kay'shuhn*). The process of thickening and hardening of the skin, often the result of repeated irritations produced by scratching or rubbing, as in eczema.

ligament. 1. A tough, flexible band of fibrous tissue that attaches to joint ends of bones and at times spreads out into a thin envelope covering the joints. 2. Certain tough bands attached to, or arising from, the lining tissue of the abdominal cavity. Examples: the ligament attaching the kneecap to the very top of the shinbone; the tough supporting bands attaching the womb, front and sides, to the walls of the lower abdomen.

ligation. The tying of veins, arteries, or ducts with a thread or cord, as catgut or silk, most commonly performed to stop the bleeding of blood vessels necessarily severed during an operation.

ligature. (*lihg'uh-choor*). A thread or cord for tying off vessels.

lightening. The falling of the head of the developing infant into the mother's pelvis that takes place about three weeks before childbirth. This is the time when the pregnant woman notices she is "carrying lower."

limp. A halting gait. An impediment in walking.

lingua. The tongue.

lipectomy (*lih-pehk'tuh-mih*). Surgical removal of fat, as of a fatty tumor, or any unusual accumulation of fat in the belly wall or in other areas of the body.

lipodystrophy (*ligh-poh-dihss'troh-fih*). A disturbance in the handling of fat by the body in which fat disappears from under the skin in many areas of the body but remains the same in others.

lipoma. A tumor, ordinarily not dangerous, made up mostly of fat.

liposarcoma. A cancerous tumor composed of undeveloped fat cells.

lithiasis (*lih-thigh'uh-sihss*). The formation of stone in the body, as gallstones, kidney stones.

litmus. A blue pigment obtained from a lichen used to determine the presence of acids and alkalies. —*blue l. paper*. Paper saturated with litmus that turns red on contact with acid. —*red l. paper*. Paper saturated with a solution of litmus colored red with acid that turns blue on contact with alkaline solutions.

liver. The largest organ in the body, weighing approximately four pounds in the adult, and situated in the right upper part of the abdomen immediately under the diaphragm. The liver is divided into two large lobes, the right and the left; and two smaller lobes, divisions of the right lobe, the *quadrate* and *caudate* lobes. On the under surface of the liver is a depression in which the gall bladder lies. The entire liver is covered by a tough coat, the *capsule*. The unit of structure of the liver is the *lobule*, each of which is composed of liver cells in close relation to the *bile ducts*, the *hepatic artery* that brings blood from the general circulation into the liver, and the *portal vein* that directs blood out from the liver. The functions of the liver are many and vital to life as a storage house for sugar, fat, protein, vitamins, and substances that have to do with blood-formation; as a manufactory of blood proteins and the precursors of substances that serve to clot the blood, and also of those that maintain it in liquid form; as a manufactory and dispenser of bile; as a birthplace and graveyard of red blood cells; as a participant in the breakdown of carbohydrates, proteins, and fats; and as a guardian against poisons, neutralizing them before they take effect.

livid. A pale, leaden, bluish color. The discoloration produced by an injury.

lobe. A rounded part or projection of an organ that is separated from other parts of the same organ by indentations or constrictions. The lungs have five lobes, three on the right and two on the left; the liver has four lobes.

lobectomy. The surgical removal of a lobe of an organ, especially the removal of a lobe of a lung.

lobotomy (*loh-bah'tuh-mih*). The cutting across of brain tissue. An operation used in the treatment of certain mental disorders.

lobule (*lahb'youl*). A small lobe or part of a lobe.

localization. 1. The determination of the area in which an injury or disease has occurred. 2. The limitation of a condition to a specific area, as a general infection that finally localizes in the lungs, or kidneys, or on the skin.

locomotion. Movement from place to place.

lockjaw. *See* TETANUS.

loin. That part of the body which is on the side and back between the lowest ribs and the very top of the pelvis.

lordosis. Curvature of the spine with the curve forward.

lues (*loo'eez*). Syphilis.

lumbago. Backache in the region of the loin.

lumbar. Pertaining to the loin.

lumbosacral. Relating to the vertebra in the low back, from below the last rib to the tail bone.

lumen. The space inside a tube; the passageway of a duct, as the space inside a vein, artery, or thermometer.

luminal. A sedative and sleep-producing drug. Another name for *phenobarbital*.

lumpy jaw. *See* ACTINOMYCOSIS.

lunate. One of the bones of the wrist, shaped like a half-moon.

lung. The organ of breathing within which oxygen is taken from the air and carbon dioxide is expelled. There are two lungs, a right and a left, situated in the chest cavity and covered by a tissue known as the *pleura*.

lupus (*loo'puhs*). A skin disease due to tuberculosis that may also affect the lining tissue, and that is characterized by the formation of lumps and proud-flesh. —*l. erythemathosus.* A skin disease often due to allergy of the small blood vessels. A red, scaly eruption consisting of patches of various sizes and forms. May be present over the entire body. The local type is often confined to a small area on the face and is not serious. The diffuse type may involve all organs of the body and result in death. —*l. vulgaris.* A slow-developing, scarring, and deforming disease involving the skin of the face, productive of small lumps. Due to tuberculosis of the skin.

luxation. A dislocation, as a dislocated shoulder joint where no break is present, but the head of the arm bone has slipped out of its socket.

lymph. The liquid found between cells and carried from this area into lymph vessels.

lymphadenitis (*lihm-faad-uh-nigh'tihss*). Inflammation of a lymph gland.

lymphadenoma (*lihm-faad-uh-noh'muh*). A tumor-like enlargement of a lymph node.

lymphadenopathy (*lihm-faad-uh-nahp'uh-thih*). Disease or enlargement of the lymph glands.

lymphatic. Relating to lymph or a vessel through which lymph flows.

lymphoblastoma. A general term for a number of cancerous conditions of the lymph glands, and others that are not certainly cancerous, as *Hodgkin's disease*.

lymphocyte. A white blood cell without granules in its protoplasm.

lysis (*ligh'sihss*). 1. The gradual disappearance of the symptoms of a disease, especially an infectious disease. 2. The gradual disappearance of fever. 3. The dissolving of a cell or tissue as the solution of red blood cells by chemical substances and various poisons.

M

macrocyte. Exceptionally large red blood cell. Seen in the blood in certain types of anemia, especially pernicious anemia.

macula (*maak'yuh-luh*). 1. A pigmented spot upon the skin. 2. A spot in the retina, the nervous tissue in the back of the eyeball, that is the area of most distinct vision.

maggot. A worm that is the young form of certain types of insect. Maggots of the bluebottle fly feed only on decayed and dead tissue. For this reason, they are successfully used by being introduced into the wound in treatment of osteomyelitis, a pus-producing, destructive infection of the bone and bone-marrow.

maize. Indian corn. It is deficient in one of the important vitamins of the B complex, *niacin*. Thus, people who are maize eaters frequently develop a deficiency disease known as *pellagra*.

malacia (*muh-lay'shih-uh*). The softening of tissue resulting from a failure of the blood supply following disease, injury, or wear and tear, as *encephalomalacia* or softening of the brain, that may occur after an injury or hardening of the arteries in the aging.

malar. Relating to the cheek or to the cheek bone.

malaria. An infectious disease caused by a single-celled microscopic form of animal life known as *plasmodium*. It is transmitted to human beings by infected anopheles mosquitoes. Malaria is characterized by fever that comes and goes, enlargement of the spleen, and the presence of the plasmodium in the blood. A typical malarial attack consists of a stage of coldness, one of heat, and one of sweating. The chill is a shaking one that jars the patient from head to toe; the fever may rise to 105°, and the sweating that comes with the fall in fever is profuse. The plasmodium enters the red blood cell, develops there, and eventually destroys it. The malarial attack develops when a large number of plasmodia destroy and escape from the red blood cells containing them. The attacks may be at regular or irregular intervals. If the attacks occur daily the malaria is called *quotidian;* if every two days *tertian;* if every three days, *quartan.* Ordinarily, the fever is entirely gone between attacks, and, in this case, the condition is known as *intermittent fever.* If any degree of fever persists between attacks, the condition is spoken of as *remittent fever.* Malaria is also designated according to the species of plasmodium that causes it; or to the organs chiefly affected; or to the symptoms most prominent, as intestinal malaria, bilious malaria.

malariologist. A specialist in the diagnosis, treatment, and control of malaria.

malformation. A deformity; an abnormal development of a part of the body, as webbed fingers, clubbed foot, humped back.

malignant. Poisonous; endangering life, as malignant cancer.

malingerer. One who pretends inability or illness.

malleolus (*muh-lee'uh-luhss*). An extension of bone having the shape of a hammerhead.   —*lateral m.* The prominent bone on the outside of the ankle. —*medial m.* The prominent bone on the inside of the ankle.

malleus (*maal'ih-uhss*). One of the tiny bones of the middle ear, shaped like a hammer, that helps transmit sound vibrations to the internal ear.

malnutrition. Improper nutrition due to bad eating habits or actual lack of food.

malposition. An abnormal position of any organ or part, as of the developing infant within the womb.

malpractice. Improper treatment given by a doctor through ignorance, carelessness, or intention.

malunion (*maal-youn'ih-uhn*). The incomplete or imperfect growing together of adjacent parts of a bone after a break. At times, callus forms very slowly or not at all and leaves the bone fragments only loosely joined.

mamma. The breast; the gland that secretes milk. —*m. virilis.* The breast of the male.

mammectomy. The surgical removal of the breast.

mammose. Having unusually large breasts.

mandible. The lower jawbone.

mania. 1. A marked excitement; a violent passion or desire. 2. A type of mental disorder characterized by a high mood with unusual feelings of well-being, delusions of greatness, and physical overactivity.

manipulation. Using the hands skillfully, as in changing the position of the developing infant within the womb, returning a bone to its joint after it has been dislocated.

manubrium (*maa-nyou'brih-uhm*). 1. A handle. 2. The top portion of the breastbone.

manus. The hand.

marasmus (*mah-raaz'muhss*). A shrinkage and gradual wasting of the body caused by a lack of, or imperfect food, or improper utilization of good food.

marrow. The soft tissue in the hollows of bone. —*red m.* Marrow that is active in forming blood cells. —*yellow m.* Marrow that no longer produces red blood cells and that, for the most part, has become fat.

marsupialization (*mahr-soo-pih-uhl-ih-zay'shuhn*). An operation performed upon a cyst of any kind when it is impossible to remove it completely. The cyst is cut open, the walls turned out, and its edges sewed to the edges of the skin incision. This wound finally heals by growth of tissue from the bottom of the cyst to the level of the skin.

masculinization. The appearance of male secondary sex characteristics in a female, as the deepening of the voice, the appearance of face hair, the thinning of head hair, the shrinking of the breasts, the accumulation of abdominal fat. Occurs in many women following the change of life.

masochism (*maaz'uh-kihsm*). Sexual deviation in which pleasure is obtained on receiving pain or cruel treatment.

massage. A type of stroking, rubbing, or kneading various parts of the body with the hands or an instrument, to relieve tension, increase circulation, break up adhesions, accelerate the return of motion, and so forth. —*buttonhole method of cardiac m.* A means of stimulating the heart to start beating after it has stopped. A small incision is made just below the lower end of the breast bone. The thumb of the right hand is pushed through the opening with the fingers under the rib margin and extended upwards. The heart can be compressed between the thumb and fingers. Repeated compression and relaxation often induces the heart to start beating again.

mastalgia (*maass-taal'jih-uh*). Pain in the breast.

mastectomy. The surgical removal of the breast.

mastication. The act of chewing.

mastitis. Inflammation of the breast. —*cystic m.* Formation of cysts in the milk ducts of the breast. These may be single or many. Most frequently occurs in childless women. —*puerperal m.* In some women, within the first three months after childbirth, a condition develops wherein the breasts become hard and painful from retention of milk.

mastoid. A small, breast-shaped protrusion of bone situated behind the ear and containing many air cells.

mastoidectomy. The surgical destruction of the air cells in the mastoid.

mastoiditis. Inflammation of the mastoid cells.

masturbation. Self-manipulation of the genital to produce a climax. Also called *chiromania, self-abuse.*

matrix. 1. The cavity in which anything is formed. 2. That section of tissue into which any organ is set, as the flesh into which a fingernail is set. 3. The substance between the cells of a tissue.

maturation. Arriving at full development.

maxilla. The bone of the upper jaw.

maxillofacial (*maak-sihl-loh-fay'shuhl*). Relating to the lower half of the face.

measles. A contagious disease, most often of childhood, that begins with a running nose, cough, inflammation of the eyes, appearance of bluish spots on the inside of the cheeks. On the third or fourth day there is usually a chill with fever and a small red eruption appears on the face or behind the ears and spreads over the body. In several days the eruption fades and is followed by scaling. The patient is sickest at the height of the eruption. One attack usually results in immunity. The disease is caused by a virus and is carried from person to person in close contact.

meatus (*mih-ay'tuhss*). An opening or passage, as the meatus of the urethra, the opening at the tip of the penis into its passageway; the auditory meatus, the ear canal.

meconium (*mih-koh'nih-uhm*). A greenish mass, pasty in consistency, that collects in the intestine of the infant developing within the womb. It is composed of mucus, bile, and other constituents. Meconium is the contents of the newborn's first bowel movement and is not entirely voided until about the fourth day of life.

media. The middle of the three coats of a vein, artery, or lymph vessel.

medial. Toward the mid-line of the body, as the nose is medial to the eye, the breast is medial to the arm.

mediastinum (*mee-dih-aas-tigh'nuhm*). 1. A separation of parts. 2. The space in the chest between the two lungs containing essentially the heart and its sac, the large arteries and veins of the body, part of the windpipe that splits into the bronchi, the gullet, the major vessel that carries lymph, various lymph glands, the thymus gland, and a few muscles.

medical examiner. 1. An officer of a state, city, or town, whose duty is to uncover facts concerning the cause of death and violent injuries, and to testify thereto in court. This office has replaced the coroner in many areas. 2. An officer whose duty is to determine facts relating to injuries and death for the corporation or bureau where he works.

medicine. 1. Any substance used to treat disease. 2. The healing art; the science of treating disease; the nonsurgical specialties in medicine.

medium. 1. That in which anything moves, or through which it acts, as the air that is the medium of man's living, the water that is the medium of other classes of life.

medulla (*mih-dul'luh*). 1. The marrow. 2. Anything that resembles marrow in its construction or in its relation to other parts, as the central parts of certain organs known as medulla in distinction to the outer parts known as *cortex*. —*m. oblongata*. The enlarged upper part of the spinal cord that connects it with the brain, the site of many vital centers, as the nervous tissue controlling breathing, the heart rate, sleep, and other important functions.

megalomania (*mehg-uh-loh-may'-nih-uh*). The delusion of personal greatness, often seen in schizophrenia where the patient acts out his ideas of his own importance.

melalgia (*meh-laal'jih-uh*). Pain in the extremities.

melancholia. A type of mental disturbance marked by fear, brooding, deep depression, and reluctance to engage in any activity. At times, however, a person so afflicted may show very definite overactivity. There are varying degrees of melancholia: mild, called *retardation;* average, called *acute depression;* severe, called *stuporous depression.*

melanin (*mehl'uh-nihn*). Black or dark-brown pigment found, in some degree, in all people and responsible for complexion. The brunette is darker than the blonde by virtue of more melanin in the skin.

melanoma (*mehl-uh-noh'muh*). A tumor that arises from a pigmented mole. Usually not serious.

melanosis (*mehl-uh-noh'sihss*). The dark-brown or black coloration of skin surfaces and lining tissues. Melanosis of the skin may be due to a type of adrenal-gland disease known as *Addison's disease.* It may also be seen in sunburn, and during pregnancy where it occurs about the nipples.

membrane. A thin layer of tissue lining a cavity, surrounding a part, connecting parts that are side by side, or separating cavities that are side by side. Examples: the lining membrane of the nose, intestinal tract, bronchial tube, gullet. —*mucous m.* The membrane that lines those cavities and passageways that, open to the air, are kept moist by the secretion of mucus. —*serous m.* A very thin membrane that lines closed cavities of the body; the membrane lining the joint cavities, abdominal cavity, the chest cavity. —*synovial m.* The membrane lining joint cavities and producing fluid in which the joint operates. —*tympanic m.* The eardrum.

menarche (*mih-nahr'kee*). The time when the menstrual periods first come on.

menhidrosis. A condition in which the menstrual flow, the monthly bleeding, is replaced by bloody sweat.

meninges (*meh-nihn'jeez*). The membranes that cover the brain and spinal cord. There are the *duramater, arachnoid,* and *piamater.*

meningioma (*meh-nihn-jih-oh'muh*). A tumor that arises from membranes covering the brain. May be located in the covering itself, or, at times, in other parts of the brain. Usually causes damage by pressure within the skull cavity rather than by spreading to other parts of the body.

meningism. 1. Irritation of the covering membranes of the brain and spinal cord during other specific diseases such as pneumonia, especially in childhood. 2. A kind of hysteria that resembles meningitis, also called *meningismus*.

meningitides (*meh-nihn-jiht'ih-deez*). A general term indicating inflammation of the lining membrane of the brain or spinal cord.

meningitis (*meh-nihn-jigh'tihss*). Inflammation of the membranes covering the brain or spinal cord due to such germs as syphilis, tuberculosis, and various viruses; also may be due to rickets, and other conditions.

meniscus (*meh-nihss'kuhss*). Used particularly to mean a crescent-shaped, normally occurring, piece of gristle in the knee joint.

menopause. The time of normal cessation of the monthly bleeding, usually between the forty-fifth and fiftieth year; also called *climacteric* and "change of life."

menorrhagia (*mehn-uh-ray'jih-uh*). An unusually heavy flow of blood during the menstrual period.

menorrhea (*mehn-uh-ree'uh*). 1. The normal flow of blood during menstruation. 2. Excessive menstruation.

menses (*mehn'seez*). The monthly discharge of blood from the vaginal canal during the childbearing life of the woman.

menstruation. The periodic bleeding from the womb occurring from puberty to menopause.

mensuration. The act of measuring.

mental. 1. Pertaining to the mind. 2. Pertaining to the chin.

mercurial. 1. Relating to, or caused by, mercury. 2. Any medication made of mercury or its salts.

mesentery (*mehs'uhn-tehr-ih*). A fold of the membrane that lines the abdominal cavity, and that attaches the intestine to the back wall of the abdomen.

metabolism. The over-all process of breaking down complex foodstuffs and substances into simple ones and of synthesizing the breakdown products of foodstuffs into complex tissue elements, all performed with the production of energy.

—*basal m.* The minimum amount of energy necessary to maintain the life processes when the body is at complete rest, in a warm atmosphere, twelve to eighteen hours after the intake of food.

metacarpus. That part of the hand between the wrist and the knuckles.

metamorphosis. A transformation or a change in structure, as the change from caterpillar to butterfly. —*sexual m.* A kind of sexual perversion in which the individual has the feelings and tastes of the opposite sex and assumes the dress and habits of that sex.

metastasis (*meh-taas′tuh-sihss*). The spread of disease from its original site to a distant one by conveyance of its cause through the blood or lymph vessels. Example: tuberculosis of the bone arising in the course of tuberculosis of the lung due to a spread of the germ from the lung through the blood stream.

metatarsalgia (*meh-tah-tahr-saal′jih-uh*). A sudden, severe, cramping, burning pain in the fore part of the sole of the foot. The pain is so severe, the shoe must be removed and the foot massaged for relief. Ordinarily occurs in one foot only and is thought to be caused by wearing shoes that are too short. Also called *Morton's foot.*

metatarsus (*meht-uh-tahr′suhss*). The part of the foot between the ankle and the beginning of the toes.

metrorrhagia (*meht-ruh-ray′jih-uh*). Bleeding from the womb not related to monthly bleeding.

microbe. A very small living organism visible only through the microscope. Applied to germs, especially those that cause disease in man.

microbiology. The science that deals with the life, actions, and nature of microscopic organism.

microcephaly (*migh-kroh-sehf′uh-lih*). An underdevelopment of the brain with a very thick skull that results in a small head, present at birth.

microfilaria (*migh-kroh-fih-laar′ih-uh*). The very young forms of the worm, *filaria*, that are sucked up by certain blood-sucking insects. Within the body of the insect these develop into a stage at which they cause disease in the humans bitten.

microglossia (*migh-kroh-glawss'ih-uh*). Unusual smallness of the tongue.

micromastia. Unusual smallness of the breasts.

midriasis (*mihd-rih-ay'sihss*). Enlargement of the pupil.

migraine (*migh'grayn*). Severe, one-sided headache that comes on in attacks and is preceded often by flashes of light before the eyes. As the headache grows in intensity, nausea and vomiting may occur, followed by drowsiness and sleep, after which the symptoms are relieved. Also called *sick headache, hemicrania.*

miliaria (*mihl-ih-aar'ih-uh*). An inflammation of the skin consisting of very tiny blisters and pimples accompanied by a tingling or pricking sensation, especially prevalent during the summer and in hot areas. Commonest in the folds of the skin. Also called *heat rash, prickly heat, strophulus, lichen tropicas,* and *miliaria rubra.*

milking. 1. The process of expressing milk from the breast by hand or mechanically. 2. The pressing of a finger along a flexible tube or duct in order to squeeze out the contents.

misopedia (*mihs-oh-pee'dih-uh*). A morbid hatred of all children, especially one's own.

mitral (*migh'truhl*). Relating to the valve between the atrium and ventricle on the left side of the heart.

mobilization. 1. The act of making a fused part movable. 2. The freeing of an organ during an operation in order to make it accessible. 3. The liberation of a substance stored in the body, as the mobilization of bile stored in the gall bladder.

molluscum. A chronic skin disease showing pulpy bumps. —*m. contagiosum.* A disease of long duration marked by the formation of squat, rounded, waxlike elevations, yellowish or pinkish, with a central depression, varying in size from a pinhead to a green pea.

monarticular. Relating to a single joint.

mongolism. A type of idiocy accompanied by a broad face, obliquely set eyes, flat or stubby nose, open mouth, fat and soft skin, and limp muscles.

moniliasis (*moh-nih-ligh'uh-sihss*). A condition brought about by infection with a fungus known as *Monilia* or *Candida*. Many parts of the body may be involved: the skin; the lining tissues; the lungs; the breathing tubes; the nails; the vagina; the gastrointestinal tract.

monocular. 1. Relating to, or affecting, one eye. 2. Having a single eyepiece as in the monocular microscope.

monocyte. A type of white blood cell normally occurring in very small numbers in the blood stream. The monocyte has no granules but does have a very large single nucleus. Increased numbers of monocytes are found in several conditions, as *glandular fever* or *infectious mononucleosis.*

monomania. A kind of mental disturbance in which the patient's actions and thoughts are permeated by one subject or one idea. Example: *paranoia* where the individual is chiefly concerned with people persecuting him.

mononucleosis (*moh-nuh-nyou-klih-oh'sihss*). A condition in which there is an increase beyond normal in the number of monocytes in the blood stream or tissue. *—infectious m.* A disease of unknown cause communicated from person to person, manifested by fever, sore throat, swollen lymph glands all over the body, especially those on the back of the neck, and an increase in the number of monocytes (some of which are of abnormal form) in the blood stream. Not uncommonly the spleen is enlarged and there may be a measles-like eruption on the skin. In its early stages, this condition is often mistaken for a childhood contagious disease or influenza. Also called *glandular fever* and *Pfeiffer's disease.*

monoplegia (*moh-nuh-plee'jih-uh*). The paralysis of a single group of muscles, as the calf muscles; or of a single limb, as an arm or leg.

mons. An anatomic prominence, an elevated area. *—m. pubis.*

The prominence in front of the body just above the genitals upon which there is a growth of hair after puberty. —*m. veneris.* The female *mons pubis.*

monster. A fetus that through faulty development is not capable of performing the vital functions; or that differs markedly from the normal human being in a deficiency of parts, an excess of parts, or an unusual formation of parts. There are many types of monsters named according to appearance (as the frog-faced monster), or according to the deformed parts. Monster births are very rare and are not the result of any fault in the parents.

monstrosity. The state of being a monster. Also, something monstrous.

morbid. Relating to diseased parts or to a disease itself, as a morbid condition meaning a condition of disease.

morbidity. 1. The character of disease or the state of being diseased. 2. The various conditions producing disease. 3. The proportion of sick people in the total population of a community.

moribund. In a dying state.

moron. An individual whose mental age is from 7 to 12 years and whose I.Q. is between 50 and 74. *See* INTELLIGENCE QUOTIENT.

morphinism (*mawr'fih-nihsm*). 1. The condition caused by addiction to morphine. 2. The morphine habit.

morphology. A subdivision of biology that deals with the form and structure of various living organisms and their parts. It includes the study of anatomy, the study of cells and their structure, and the development of parts.

mortal. Deadly; ending in death; causing death; liable to disintegration or death.

motile. Capable of movement; able to move as certain germs that propel themselves.

motion. 1. The act of changing places. 2. A movement of the bowels; the matter excreted from the bowels. —*passive m.* Movement produced in an individual by an agency other than himself. For example, the movement of the leg and arms made in the process of certain types of massage, to help recovery of function after a bone fracture.

motion sickness. A general term that includes air sickness, car sickness, seasickness, characterized by dizziness, nausea, vomiting as a result of motion of a ship, airplane, automobile, train, or any other moving vehicle in which the patient is riding.

motor. 1. That which produces motion. 2. Concerned in, or pertaining to, motion, as the nerves that transmit impulses that result in the movement of a muscle, called *motor nerves.*

mountain sickness. A condition that occurs at very high altitudes, especially over fifteen thousand feet, caused by a reduction in air pressure that exists at this altitude. The symptoms are loss of appetite, nausea, vomiting, rapid and difficult breathing, weakness, a bluing of the lips and skin, headache, very rapid heart rate; or, at times, an unusual feeling of well-being.

mouth. 1. The beginning of the digestive tube; the cavity in which chewing takes place. At times used in a less general sense to indicate the opening of the lips. 2. The entrance to any body cavity or canal.

movement. The act of moving. —*active m.* Movement produced by the individual himself without any outside help, as lifting an arm, walking, chewing. —*ciliary m.* Many cells, particularly those composing the lining tissue of the nose, throat, and bronchial tubes, have tiny hairlike extensions from their border. These are called *cilia.* These cilia have a whiplike movement whose function is to move particles of matter of any kind in one or another direction. —*fetal m.* The movement of the developing infant within the womb, felt by the mother as shoving and pushing against the belly wall. —*passive m.* Movement produced in an individual or organism by some outside factor.

mucin (*myou'sihn*). A certain type of protein that forms the base of mucus. Mucus is produced by the lining tissue of many hollow organs such as the nose, bronchial tubes, stomach, and intestines. When produced by the bronchial tubes, it is commonly called *phlegm*.

mucocutaneous (*myou-koh-kyou-tay'nih-uhss*). Relating to the line at which mucous membrane and skin meet, as the meeting of the skin and mucous membrane where the red begins on the lips.

mucosa (*myou-koh'suh*). Another name for mucous membrane; a lining tissue that produces mucus.

mucous (*myou'kuhss*). Pertaining to mucus; producing mucus, as a mucous gland, many of which are found in the lining tissue of hollow organs.

mucus (*myou'kuhss*). A thick liquid produced and expelled by special glands known as mucous glands, consisting of water, mucin, salts, and certain sloughed-off cells. Mucus keeps moist the various lining tissues of the body's hollow organs.

multigravida (*mul-tih-graav'ih-duh*). A pregnant woman who has had two or more pregnancies in the past.

mumps. A communicable disease of sudden onset, caused by a virus. Most often occurs in childhood, one attack usually giving a lifelong immunity. The symptoms are swelling of the large gland that produces saliva, situated in the face below the ear, and (at times) other salivary glands in the floor of the mouth as well as (at times) the testicles, ovaries, and pancreas. The time between the reception of the virus by an individual and the appearance of symptoms is approximately three weeks, when there is pain and swelling below the ear with fever. At the end of a week the swelling begins to disappear. No pus is produced.

mural. Relating to a wall, as the wall of the heart, the womb, a blood vessel, the stomach, as mural fibroids, mural abscess, mural thrombus.

murmur. A sound heard through the stethoscope in the region of the heart or blood vessels that is abnormal and usually has a blowing or rasping quality.

muscle. A tissue that shortens by contracting and lengthens by relaxing and that, by virtue of this alternating state, moves organs or parts of the body. Thus the opposite ends of a muscle attached to the bones on either side of a joint will cause the movement of the joint through this alternating contraction and relaxation. Muscles are classified according to their appearance under a microscope. Seen under great magnification, some muscle fibers show a pronounced horizontal striping. These are called *striped* muscles and are under the control of the will. Others show a faint horizontal striping. These are found only in the heart and are not under the control of the will. Still others show no stripe at all. These, called *unstriped* muscles, are not under the control of the will and are found in the intestine, womb, bladder, blood-vessels, and so on. Muscles are further classified according to their relation to the will as *voluntary* and *involuntary*; according to location, as heart, skeletal, intestinal, and so on.

mutism. The state of being speeechless; dumbness. —*hysterical m.* Mutism that is due to a mental or emotional state. This condition was seen frequently during the last war in soldiers who experienced a severe emotional shock in battle. It is also seen in schizophrenia. The vocal organs are perfectly normal in these cases.

myalgia (*migh-aal'jih-uh*). Pain in the muscles, such as in rheumatism.

myasthenia (*migh-aass-thee'nih-uh*). Great muscular weakness. —*m. gravis pseudoparalytica.* A disease of unknown cause in which the voluntary muscles, those under the control of the will, become exhausted very rapidly. May become a very serious condition since it may affect the muscles of swallowing and breathing.

myatonia (*migh-uh-toh'nih-uh*). A state of limpness of the muscles. —*m. congenita.* Myatonia that appears in infants and affects only the muscles of the trunk, extremities, abdominal wall.

mycology. The science that deals with fungi.

mycosis. Any infection caused by a fungus. Mycosis may be superficial, as in *barber's itch* involving the skin of the face; or it may be internal.

myectomy. The surgical removal of a piece of muscle.

myelin (*migh'uh-lihn*). A sheath of white, fatty substance covering some nerves.

myelitis (*migh-eh-ligh'tihss*). 1. Inflammation of the spinal cord. 2. Inflammation of bone marrow.

myelogram (*migh'eh-loh-graam*). An X-ray of the spinal cord and canal made after the introduction of air or iodine-containing oils into the spinal canal. These latter substances serve to outline the spinal canal and its various spaces on the X-ray film.

myeloma (*migh-eh-loh'muh*). A tumor of the bone marrow, threatening to life.

myocarditis. An inflammation of the muscular wall of the heart.

myocardium. The muscle that makes up the heart.

myoclonus (*migh-oh-kloh'nuhss*). Spasms of a muscle, or a number of muscles, occurring one after another in rhythm.

myoma. A tumor that arises from muscle. When it comes from smooth muscle, that is, unstriped muscle, it is called *leiomyoma*; when it comes from striped muscle, it is called *rhabdomyoma*.

myomectomy (*migh-oh-mehk'tuh-mih*). The surgical removal of a muscle tumor, as the tumors of the womb wall.

myopathy (*migh-ahp'uh-thih*). Any disease of the muscles, as rheumatism.

myopia. Nearsightedness, due to a greater than normal length of the eyeball from front to back, resulting in the image falling in front of the retina. Lenses similar to reducing lenses that push the image back onto the retina are used to correct this condition.

myosis. The constriction of the pupil of the eye.

myositis. Inflammation of muscle, usually of muscle under the control of the will.

myotonia. Continuous spasm of muscles not relieved by relaxation. —*m. congenita.* A disease occurring at birth, probably hereditary, characterized by unrelieved spasms of the muscles under the control of the will. Also known as *Thomsen's disease.*

myringitis (*mihr-ihn-jigh'tihss*). Inflammation of the eardrum.

myringodectomy (*mihr-ihn-goh-dehk'tuh-mih*). The surgical removal of part or all of the eardrum.

myringotome (*mihr-ihn'goh-tohm*). A surgical instrument used for cutting into the eardrum.

myringotomy (*mihr-ihn-gaht'uh-mih*). The cutting into the eardrum.

myxedema (*mihk-seh-dee'muh*). A condition usually occurring after childhood due to a decrease in the amount of thyroid hormone. This ailment may result from a shrinkage of the thyroid gland, its surgical removal, some defect in the pituitary gland that normally induces the thyroid to secrete its hormone, a difficulty in the use of thyroid hormone by the body. Myxedema is characterized by a puffy appearance, especially of the face and hands with an underlying sallowness, dryness of the skin, absence of sweating, thinning and drying of the hair, brittleness of the nails, low grade intelligence, thick and coarse speech, unusual sensitivity to cold, very slow pulse, at times a widening of the heart, and a low basal metabolism with a rate of minus 25 to minus 40. All degrees of this condition may appear. It is completely controlled by the proper amount of thyroid given by mouth or injection. Also called *Gull's disease.*

N

nail. The hornlike plate that covers the ends of the fingers and toes composed of the horny layer of skin cells. —*n. bed*. The tissue upon which the nail rests, consisting of many small blood vessels.

nail biting. A manifestation of nervousness in children and young adolescents who bite the fingernails down to the quick. Often it is difficult to break this habit, which may persist into middle age unless the underlying emotional disturbance is uncovered. Also called *onychophagia*.

narcissism (*nahr′sihss-ihsm*). Self-love, often without sexuality involved. This term is derived from a Greek myth of a beautiful youth, Narcissus, who fell in love with his own reflection.

narcolepsy. A condition characterized by attacks of deep sleep that last for a very short time. May be caused by epilepsy, inflammation of the brain, and tumors in the brain stem. Is serious only because of what may occur during the sleep attacks, as falling asleep while crossing the street or driving an automobile.

narcosis. A condition of unconsciousness, arrested activity, or deep stupor, the result of medication or disease.

narcosynthesis. A type of treatment used in psychoneurosis, especially in neurosis that arises out of a war situation. A drug, as sodium amytal, is injected into the vein of the patient, producing a state of semi-sleep during which the patient is induced to talk of the episode causing the neurosis. This revelation is discussed with him in a waking state, usually with excellent results.

narcotic. 1. Having the quality of producing a deep unconsciousness. 2. Any drug that produces sleep, insensibility, or stupor. There are three main groups: *the opium group*, that induces sleep; the *alcohol group*, that produces exhilaration and sleep; the *belladonna group*, that produces illusions and delirium. 3. An individual with the narcotic habit.

narcotize. To make unconscious or put under the influence of a narcotic.

naris (*naar'ihss*). A nostril. One of a pair of openings at the front part of the nose, or at the back part of the nose where it opens into the space above the throat.

nasal. 1. (*adj.*) Relating to the nose. 2. (*n.*) The bone that forms the bridge of the nose.

nasopharynx (*nay-zoh-faar'ihnks*). The space behind the nose in the throat above the level of the roof of the mouth.

nasus (*nay'zuhss*). The nose.

nausea. An uncomfortable feeling in and about the stomach associated with an aversion for food and a need to vomit.

navicular (*nuh-vihk'yuh-luhr*). 1. Boat-shaped. 2. A bone of the wrist and the ankle.

near point. The point nearest the eye at which an object can be seen distinctly.

Necator (*nih-kay'tuhr*). A type of hookworm. —*n. americanus*. The type of hookworm prevalent throughout the tropics of the western hemisphere and the southern United States.

necatoriasis (*neh-kuh-tuh-righ'uh-sihss*). Infestation with the American hookworm. The egg enters the skin through the webs of the fingers and toes. In the last century when going barefoot was so common in certain depressed areas of the South, hookworm was rampant. Once in the blood stream, the egg finds its way into the small intestine and may do damage here and in the lungs.

neck. 1. The narrow part of the body connecting the head with the trunk. 2. A narrow part of any structure or organ serving to join its parts, as the neck of the bladder, the neck of the gall bladder.

necromania. A morbid desire for death or an unusual attraction to dead bodies.

necrophilism. A sexual perversion in which intercourse is had with dead bodies.

necropsy (*nehk'rahp-sih*). An autopsy; an examination of a body after death.

necrosis. The death of a cell, group of cells, or a tissue that is in contact with or surrounded by living cells or tissues. —*caseation n*. Occurring particularly in tuberculosis, the formation of a cheesy substance in the tissue destroyed by the germ. —*ischemic n*. The death of tissue due to the blockage of an artery supplying it. Often happens when the artery of the heart is blocked with a clot.

needling. A surgical procedure in which a needle is used to tear a tissue, as the operation performed for cataract, where a needle is inserted into the lens of the eye, the site of the cataract. The outer covering of the lens is torn to permit the passage of the lens material into the front chamber of the eye. This action results in a clearing of the cataract.

Neisseria (*nigh-see'rih-uh*). A kind of germ to which belong the organisms that cause gonorrhea and epidemic meningitis.

Nematoda (*nehm-uh-toh'duh*). A general group of worms; the true round worms. May cause disease in man.

nematology. The study of nematode worms.

neonatorum (*nee-oh-nuh-taw'ruhm*). Relating to the newborn.

neoplasm. Any new growth, as a tumor.

nephrectomy. The surgical removal of a kidney.

nephritis. Inflammation of the kidney. May be caused by a number of conditions or follow on such diseases as scarlet fever. Included in this class of disease is *Bright's disease*.

nephrolithiasis (*nehf-roh-lih-thigh'uh-sihss*). The formation of stones in the kidney or the disease condition that leads to their formation.

nephrolithotomy (*nehf-roh-lih-thaht'uh-mih*). Surgical cutting of a kidney for the removal of stone.

nephroma. A tumor of the outer portion of the kidney of serious nature, dangerous to life, common in adults.

nephropexy. The sewing into place of a floating kidney.

nephrosclerosis. A kidney condition that comes on in cases of high blood pressure, eventually producing symptoms of *Bright's disease*. A form, *malignant n.*, is a rapid and progressively serious condition of the kidneys that often results in death.

nephrosis. Disintegration of the kidney without signs of inflammation. —*acute n.* A condition that follows or accompanies an infectious disease or poisoning, as with mercury. —*chronic lipoid n.* A condition frequently seen in children where there is some inability of the body to properly handle proteins, characterized especially by albumen and fat droplets in the urine. —*chronic n.* A condition of slow kidney disintegration associated with diseases of metabolism, as diabetes or gout.

nephrotomy (*neh-fraht-uh-mih*). The surgical cutting into the kidney.

nerve. A bundle of nervous fibers that exist usually outside of the brain and spinal cord. The nerve fibers are like large and small cables and are held together by an outer sheath and by inner tough, connecting tissue. Such a cable of nerve fibers within the brain or the spinal cord is called a *nerve tract*. The nerves are transmission wires of sensation from the outer world to the brain and spinal cord, and of stimuli from the brain and spinal cord to various areas and specialized tissues, causing them to act (as voluntary motion), or for the production of special substances (as digestive juices when food is taken into the mouth).

nervous system. The entire nervous structure of the body including the *brain* and its *stem*; the *spinal cord*; the various *nerves* and their relay stations, the *ganglia*. There are two major divisions: the *central nervous system*, that generally governs volition; the *autonomic nervous system*, that generally governs activity over which the will has no control, as the functioning of the stomach and intestine, the secretion of glands.

neural. Relating to nerves or nervous tissue.

neuralgia. Severe attacks of sharp, stabbing pain of short duration and tenderness along the course of a nerve in any part of the body. Not due to disease of the nerve itself.

neurasthenia (*nyou-raas-thee'nih-uh*). A condition caused by emotional disturbance and manifested by lack of energy, readiness to fatigue, a reluctance to engage in any activity, various aches, and pains. Symptoms vary, being referable to the entire body in some individuals and localized in one region or organ in others.

neuritis. Inflammation of a nerve or nerves. Symptoms are excessive sensitivity, pain, paralysis, loss of sensitivity, numbness and tingling, and shrinkage of the muscles supplied by the involved nerve. Symptoms vary according to the nerve involved and the severity of the affection.

neurodermatitis (*nyou-roh-duhr-muh-tigh'tihss*). A disorder of the skin in which thickened and itchy patches appear (often in the same position) on both sides of the body, usually on the neck, in the bend of the elbow, the bend of the knee. It is related to emotional disturbance.

neurofibromatosis (*nyou-roh-figh-broh-muh-toh'sihss*). A condition in which many tumors are present in the skin along the course of nerves, usually painless but occasionally threatening to life. Also called *von Recklinghausen's disease, Molluscum fibrosum.*

neurogenic. 1. Arising from nerves, as a neurogenic tumor. 2. Stimulated through the nervous system, as muscle spasms.

neurologist. A physician who specializes in the treatment and recognition of disorders of the nervous system.

neuron. The total nerve cell that includes the *body of the cell* and the *dendrites*, long hairlike processes that transmit impulses into the body of the cell, and an *axon*, a conductor of impulses from the body of the cell outward.

neuropathy (*nyou-rahp-uh-thih*). Any disease of the nervous system.

neuropsychiatry. That specialty in medicine that deals with nervous and mental diseases.

neuroretinitis (*nyou-roh-reht-ih-nigh'tihss*). Inflammation of both the nerve of vision and the retina.

neurosis. *See* PSYCHONEUROSIS.

neurosurgeon. A specialist in surgery of the brain and nervous system.

neutrophil (*nyou'troh-fihl*). A type of white blood cell with granules in its protoplasm that stain with neutral dye.

nevus (*nee'vuhss*). 1. A birthmark. 2. A small area on the skin, pigmented or containing many small blood vessels, that appears at, or shortly after, birth. 2. A tumor of the skin composed of blood vessels.

nictitation. Excessive winking.

nidation (*nigh-day'shuhn*). The implantation of an egg that has been penetrated by a sperm into the lining tissue of the womb.

night blindness. Defective night vision. When temporary may be due to a deficiency of vitamin A. When permanent may be due to diseases of the retina, as *retinitis pigmentosa*. Also called *nyctalopia*.

night cry. A piercing cry of a child during sleep. Most often of psychological origin; at times indicative of physical disease, as an early stage of hip disease.

night pain. Pain occurring in a limb during sleep at the time when the muscles are relaxed. Often occurs in the hip or knee and may be a symptom of hip disease.

night palsy (*pawl'zih*). Tingling and numbness of the arms and legs occurring during the night, or on waking in the morning, often affecting women during the change of life.

nipple. The cone-shaped projection in the middle of the

breast that contains the exits of the milk tubes. Also called *papilla*.

nocturia. 1. Bed wetting at night. 2. The need to pass water frequently at night.

node. 1. A small rounded knob. 2. A point of constriction. —*singer's n.* A small protuberance on the vocal cord often found in people who use their voices a great deal.

nodule. 1. A small node. 2. A small group of cells.

normocyte. A red blood cell of normal size.

normocytosis A normal condition of the cells of the blood.

nose. The organ in the center of the face, between the eyes. In the upper interior part are the organs of smell; in the lower part, inhaled air is warmed, moistened, and cleared of its impurities.

nosology. The science of classification of diseases.

nostomania. Homesickness of such a degree that it becomes a monomania.

notifiable. Relating to a disease that must be reported to health authorities, as scarlet fever or chicken pox.

noxious. Harmful; causing ill effects; poisonous.

nubile (*nyou'bihl*). Of an age for childbearing.

nucha (*nyou'kuh*). The nape of the neck.

nullipara (*nuhl-lihp'uh-ruh*). A woman who has never had a child.

nummular (*num'you-luhr*). Resembling a coin or roll of coins in form. Used particularly to describe a certain skin disease in which the eruption is shaped like a coin or many coins.

nutrition. 1. All of the processes that are involved in the growth, maintenance, and repair of the body. 2. Food or nourishment.

nyctalope (*nihk'tuh-lohp*). One who cannot see at night.

nyctaphobia. An unnatural fear of night and darkness.

nymphectomy. The surgical removal of one or both of the small lips of the vagina.

nymphomania. Excessive sexual need on the part of a woman.

nystagmus (*nih-staag'muhss*). Rapid movements of the eyeball with return to the normal position, occurring in series. It can be exhibited best if one watches an individual looking out of the window of a rapidly moving train. The eyes travel back and forth with great rapidity. The movement may be to one side or the other, up and down, around. Nystagmus may be due to disease or it may be due to some defect existing at birth.

O

obesity. A condition in which excessive fat is accumulated in the body. May be glandular or due to overeating, often a manifestation of psychological disturbances.

obliteration. 1. The complete surgical removal of a part, or its destruction by disease. 2. Closure of a cavity or passageway. 3. Total loss of memory, or awareness of certain events.

obsession. An emotion or an idea that continues in a person's mind despite all attempts to remove it.

obstetrician. A medical specialist who cares for women during pregnancy, labor, and the three-month period when the womb returns to normal.

obstruction. A state of being obstructive; a blockage in a hollow organ, a tube, or a blood vessel. —*intestinal o.* Any obstacle to the passage of the bowel contents. —*ureteral o.* Any blockage of the flow of urine from the kidney through the ureter to the bladder. —*urinary o.* Any blockage to the passage of urine from the bladder out.

obturator (*ahb'tyuh-ray-tuhr*). 1. A solid wire or thin rod used to block the passageway of a needle. This rod usually is pointed and extends to the tip of the needle. Its purpose is twofold; it makes for a firmer piercing instrument and permits the control of the flow of fluid from the vein, spinal canal, or other hollow organ into which the needle is inserted. 2. The name of certain muscles. 3. An appliance that closes a split in the palate (roof of the mouth).

occipital (*ahk-sihp'ih-tuhl*). Relating to the bone that constitutes the back part of the head.

occiput (*ahk'sih-puht*). The back part of the head.

occlusion. 1. A shutting or closing. 2. The condition of being shut. 3. In dentistry, the full meeting (when in a position of rest) of the chewing surfaces of the upper and lower teeth.

occult. Not evident. Hidden, as blood, not visible to the eye, in the contents of bowel evacuation proved to be present by certain tests.

occupational disease. Disease caused by the patient's occupation, due either to the work itself, to the materials used in the work, or to the atmosphere in which the work is done. Examples: *anthracosis,* a blackening and inflammation of the lungs occurring in coal miners due to the inhalation of soft coal dust; *lead colic,* occurring in painters due to the white lead in the paint.

occupational therapy. A type of adjunct treatment in which ability and interest are developed in particular arts or trades for those who are handicapped physically or mentally.

octigravida (*ahk-tih-graav'ih-duh*). A woman who is pregnant for the eighth time.

octipara (*ahk-tihp'uh-ruh*). A woman who has been in labor eight times.

ocular. 1. (adj.) Relating to the eye. 2. (n.) The lens of a microscope or other optical instruments nearest to the eye; an eyepiece.

oculomotor (*ahk-yuh-loh-moh'tuhr*). Relating to the movement of the eye, or to the nerve by that name that controls some of the muscles of the eye.

odontoma. A tumor that arises from the same tissue from which teeth are formed.

oedipus complex (*ehd'ih-puhss*). A key Freudian term,

named after the central character in the play *Oedipus Rex* by Sophocles, based on Greek mythology, in which young Oedipus, prince of Thebes, brought up as a shepherd and ignorant of his descent, slays his father and marries his mother. In all individuals in the infantile stage there is a desire to displace the parent of the same sex and to possess sexually the parent of the opposite sex. This desire comes into conflict with the reality relationship between child and parents, and as a result is pushed down below the level of awareness into the unconscious and thus repressed completely. The universal horror of incest can be traced to this repression. A positive reflection of the repressed idea may be marriage with an individual who resembles the loved parent, or repugnance toward individuals who closely resemble the unconsciously hated parent. When this repression is not accomplished in the normal manner, the foundation is laid for mental, emotion and character illnesses.

Oidium (*oh-ihd'ih-uhm*). A class of fungi that resembles both yeasts and molds. These may produce disease in man involving many parts of the body.

ointment. A medical preparation, semisolid in character, used to protect or soothe the skin, or as a base for various types of medicine. The essential constituents of ointments are mixtures of fats, waxes, and vegetable, animal, and/or mineral oils, or a water emulsion.

olecranon (*oh-lehk'ruh-nahn*). The prominent, bony extension on the inner part of the elbow.

oleothorax. Compression of the lung by the use of oil in order to maintain it at rest. Performed in tuberculosis.

oliguria (*ohl-ih-goo'rih-uh*). A lessening in the amount of urine expelled.

omentum. A fold of the tissue that lines the abdominal cavity connecting the organs within this cavity to the stomach; literally means an apron.

omphalitis (*ahm-fah-ligh'tihss*). Inflammation of the navel.

omphalos (*ahm'fuh-luhss*). The navel.

onanism (*oh'nuh-nihsm*). 1. The practice of complete sexual intercourse with the discharge of semen taking place outside the vagina. 2. Masturbation.

onocology (*ahn-oh-kahl-uh-jih*). The science embracing tumor growth.

onomatomania (*ahn-uh-maa-tuh-may'nih-uh*). A compulsion to repeat certain words.

onychia (*oh-nihk'ih-uh*). Inflammation of the tissue under the nails.

onychomycosis (*ahn-ih-koh-migh-koh'sihss*). A fungus disease of the nails.

onychophagia. *See* NAIL BITING.

onyx. 1. A finger- or toenail. 2. An accumulation of pus, shaped like a fingernail, in the anterior chamber of the eye.

oophorectomy (*oh-oh-faw-rehk'tuh-mih*). The surgical removal of an ovary.

oophoritis (*oh-oh-faw-righ'tihss*). Inflammation of an ovary.

opacity. 1. The state of not permitting light to pass through. 2. A spot on the transparent part of the eye, or in the lens, that does not permit light to pass through.

operable. A condition that can be relieved by operation.

operation. Any procedure performed on the living person; a procedure performed by a surgeon with instruments by a definite method. —*elective o.* One in which the time for surgery can be set in advance, as removal of adenoids or tonsils, reshaping the nose, and other plastic operations. —*emergency o.* One that must be done immediately in order to save the patient's life or to prevent the disease from spreading. —*exploratory o.* One done in order to establish a diagnosis, to discover what is actually wrong. —*major o.* One in which the risk to life is considerable, as most operations in which the abdominal cavity is opened. —*minor o.* One in which there is little or no danger to life. —*radical o.* One in which not only the cause of the condition is removed but in which enough tissue is removed so that chances for future return of the condition are minimal. —*reconstructive* *o.* One in which a defect is repaired, as a broken nose, a harelip.

ophthalmia (*ahf-thaal'mih-uh*). Inflammation of the eye, particularly where the lining tissue of the eye and lids is involved. —*catarrhal o.* Inflammation of the lining membrane of the eye with reddening and the presence of mucus and pus. —*o. neonatorum.* Inflammation of the eye in the newborn due to gonorrhea or other acute infections. To prevent or cure this, silver nitrate drops are routinely put into the eyes of newborn infants. —*phlyctenular o.* A small, blistery inflammation of the lining tissue of the eyeball and the transparent part of the eye caused by tuberculosis in childhood. —*sympathetic o.* Severe inflammation of an eye following injury to the opposite eye.

ophthalmic (*ahf-thaal'mihk*). Relating to the eye.

ophthalmologist (*ahf-thaal-mahl-uh-jihst*). A specialist in the eye and its diseases.

ophthalmology. The science of the structure, function, and diseases of the eye.

ophthalmoplegia (*ahf-thaal-moh-plee'jih-uh*). Paralysis of the muscles of the eye.

ophthalmoscope. An instrument for examining the interior of the eye consisting of a searchlight, the light rays of which are concentrated in a small point and directed into the pupil, and small magnifying lenses through which the examiner looks.

opiate. Any preparation of opium, as laudanum, paregoric, opium itself, morphine.

optic. Relating to the eye.

optician. One who makes lenses or optical instruments. —*dispensing o.* One who sells spectacles.

optometrist. One who measures the seeing ability without the use of eyedrops.

oral. Relating to the mouth.

oral erotism. Sexual excitation from stimulation of the lips or mouth as seen in kissing or various perversions.

orbicular. Circular. Applied to muscles arranged in circles, as the muscle around the mouth (*orbicularis oris*).

orbit. The eyesocket; formed by seven bones.

orchic. Relating to the testes.

orchiectomy (*awr-kih-ehk'tuh-mih*). The surgical removal of one or both testes.

orchiopexy (*awr-kih-oh-pehk'sih*). The surgical fixing of a testis into the scrotum performed where the testis has not descended completely into the scrotal sac.

orchis (*awr'kihs*). Testis. Male sex gland.

orchitis (*awr-kigh'tihss*). Inflammation of the testis.

orgasm. The peak of excitement during sexual intercourse culminating in the ejaculation of semen in the male, and in relaxation in the female.

ornithosis. A disease found in birds, particularly pigeons and domestic fowl, due to a virus that at times causes pneumonia in man.

oropharynx. The throat above the voice box and below the level of the soft palate.

orthopedics. A surgical specialty that deals with correction of deformities and diseases of muscles, joints, and bones.

orthopedist. A specialist in orthopedics.

orthopsychiatry. A branch of psychiatry concerned essentially with the prevention and treatment of behavior disorders. Mental hygiene is one of the main interests of orthopsychiatry.

orthoptics. The science that deals with the correction of faulty sight by means of exercise or training, as treatment of the lack of muscle balance in cases of crossed eyes.

os[1] (*ahss*). The mouth. Applied to the opening of certain organs, as the womb.

os[2] (*ahss*). A bone, as *os calcis*, the heel bone; *os coxae*, the hip bone.

oscillometer (*ahs-sih-lahm'ih-tuhr*). An instrument for measuring swings, vibrations, or any tremulous motion, as a blood pressure machine.

oscitation (*ahs-sih-tay′shuhn*). The act of yawning.

osmosis. The passing of a fluid through a membrane in the direction of a more concentrated fluid, as in the expansion of a prune or dried apricot when placed in water due to water passing into the fruit by osmosis.

osseous (*ahs′sih-uhss*). Bony; made of, or resembling bone.

ossicle. A small bone, particularly one of three small bones in the middle ear.

ossification. The formation of bone, or the change of tissue into bone.

ossify. Turn into bone.

osteitis (*ahs-tee-igh′tihss*). Inflammation of bone as the result of infections like syphilis, or overactivity of the parathyroids, one of the endocrine glands. The latter condition, known as *osteitis fibrosa cystica*, is characterized by thinning of all the bones in the body, and formation of large cysts.

osteocarcinoma (*ahs-tih-uh-kahr-sih-noh′muh*). Cancer of the bone.

osteochondritis (*ahs-tih-uh-kahn-drigh′tihss*). Inflammation involving both bone and gristle from which bone is formed. —*o. deformans juvenilis.* Inflammation of the upper thigh bone, especially in children between five and ten. Also called *Legg-Calve-Perthes′ disease, coxa plana.* —*o. dissecans.* Gristle normally covers the ends of bones within joints; in *o. dissecans* a piece of gristle and the bone underneath it are detached and free in the joint. Most common in the knee.

osteochondroma. A tumor that arises from bone or gristle, not dangerous to life but tending to come back after surgical removal.

osteology (*ahs-tih-ahl′uh-jih*). The study of bones, their structure, and function.

osteoma. A tumor composed of various parts of bone.

osteomalacia (*ahs-tih-uh-muh-lay′shih-uh*). The softening of bone with resulting deformities, usually due to a deficiency in vitamin D with loss of calcium. Occurs mostly in pregnant women.

ostium. A mouth or opening, as *ostium vaginae*, the outer opening of the vagina.

otic. Pertaining to the ear.

otitis. Inflammation of the ear. —*o. externa.* Inflammation of the external ear. —*o. interna.* Inflammation of the internal ear. —*o. media.* Inflammation of the middle ear.

otolaryngologist (*oh-toh-laar-uhn-gahl'uh-jihst*). A specialist in the structure, function and diseases of ear, nose, and throat.

otolaryngology. A specialty including the ear, nose, throat, and also the use of endoscope instruments, as the bronchoscope.

otologist. A specialist in the ear, its diseases, and treatment.

otosclerosis. A condition caused by the laying down of new bone around the internal ear, resulting in a progressive loss of hearing.

otoscope. An instrument for the examination of the ear and the drum.

ovarian. Relating to the ovaries.

ovariectomy (*oh-vaa-rih-ehk'tuh-mih*). The surgical removal of an ovary.

ovary (*oh'vuh-rih*). The female gland that produces the ova or egg cells that, after being penetrated by sperm, develop into new individuals. There are two ovaries, one on either side of the lower abdominal cavity.

oviduct (*oh'vih-dukt*). A tube that forms the passageway for the egg cells from the ovary to the womb; commonly called the "tubes"; known as the *Fallopian tubes.*

ovulation (*ahv-yuh-lay'shuhn*). The escape of the egg cell from the ovary occurring in humans midway between menstrual periods.

ovum. An egg cell, capable of developing into a new individual after being penetrated by the sperm.

oxygen tent. A plastic tent enclosing the head and shoulders of the patient into which oxygen is introduced and maintained at a higher concentration than that of the surrounding air.

ozena (*oh-zee'nuh*). A disease of the nose characterized by a foul discharge. Due to infection, or shrinkage of the lining membrane of the nose.

P

pachyblepharon (*paak-ih-blehf'uh-ruhn*). Thickening of the eyelid.

pachycephaly (*paak-ih-sehf'uh-lih*). Abnormal thickness of the walls of the skull.

pachydermia (*paak-ih-duhr'mih-uh*). Unusual thickening of the skin.

pachymeningitis (*paak-ih-mehn-ihn-jigh'tihss*). Inflammation of the outermost covering of the brain and spinal cord, caused by infections of syphilis or other diseases, or by long-standing bleeding within the brain.

pachyonychia (*paak-ih-oh-nihk'ih-uh*). Thickening of the nails.

pack. A dry or wet, hot or cold blanket wrapped about the body.

packing. 1. The filling of a cavity or wound with gauze or other material. 2. The material so used.

pain. 1. A sensation that causes suffering or distress. 2. Rhythmic spasm of the womb during labor. —*after p.* The painful spasm of the womb after childbirth caused by clots of blood or parts of the afterbirth remaining in the womb. —*bearing-down p.* A feeling of dragging in the low abdomen that occurs in labor and certain inflammations of the low abdominal cavity. —*false p.* Mild cramps in the abdomen that come on late in pregnancy but are not actual labor pains. —*girdle p.* Painful sensation about the waist resembling the squeezing pressure of a tight belt usually resulting from disease of the spinal cord. —*growing p.* Soreness in muscles and joints, frequently around puberty, and often an evidence of rheumatism. —*intermenstrual p.* Pain, frequently sharp and stabbing, that occurs between menstrual periods due to rupture of an ovum from the ovary. —*phantom limb p.* Pain in the area of a limb that has been amputated. —*referred p.* Pain that does not arise from any disturbance in the area where it is felt, as pain in the neck or the shoulder resulting from affection of the upper covering of the diaphragm.

painter's colic. *See* PLUMBISM.

palate (*paal'iht*). The roof of the mouth consisting of the front hard palate composed of bones covered by lining tissue, and the back soft palate made up of muscles covered by lining tissue. —*cleft p.* In the development of the palate in the fetus the two sides grow together and meet in the middle. At times this closure does not occur and a cleft or split remains that may involve the soft palate alone, or the soft and hard palate together. Cleft palate may be associated with a cleft lip, or harelip.

palatoplegia (*paal-uh-toh-plee'jih-uh*). Paralysis of the soft palate.

palliative. 1. Relieving or reducing pain or suffering. 2. A drug that soothes symptoms without curing the disease causing it.

pallor. Paleness of the skin and lining tissues.

palm. The hollow of the hand.

palpable. Capable of being touched or felt.

palpation. A method used in examinations to aid in making a diagnosis. The hand is placed upon the part of the body in question for the purpose of determining its condition or the condition of underlying organs, as palpation of the liver, spleen, or kidneys.

palpebra (*paal'pih-bruh*). *pl.* palpebrae. The eyelid. —*p.*

inferior. The lower eyelid. —*p. superior.* The upper eyelid.

palpitation. A throbbing, bumping, or fluttering, particularly of the heart; any action of the heart of which the patient is aware.

palsy (*pawl'zih*). Paralysis. —*Bell's p.* Paralysis of one side of the face with a drooping of the lid and the corner of the mouth. —*birth p.* Paralysis due to an injury of the infant during birth commonly resulting in inability to lift the arm from the side. Also called *Erb-Duchenne syndrome.* —*cerebral p.* Also called cerebral paralysis. See PARALYSIS. —*crutch p.* Paralysis of the arm due to pressure in the armpit. —*drummer's p.* Paralysis of the last segment of the thumb occurring in drummers. —*hod-carrier's p.* Because of the sustained muscular effort in holding the arms above the shoulders, or from carrying heavy loads on the shoulders, the nerve that supplies the shoulder blade is injured, resulting in the shoulder blade sticking out like a small wing. Also called *winged scapula.* —*lead p.* Due to lead poisoning, the wrist and/or ankle may hang limp through paralysis. —*printer's p.* A paralysis due to injury of many nerves on poisoning with antimony used in making type-castings. —*shaking p.* A condition, usually coming in later life, due to hardening of the arteries in a certain part of the brain. Also called *paralysis agitans, Parkinson's disease.* —*spinal p.* See PARALYSIS.

panarthritis. Inflammation of all the parts of a joint, inside and out.

pancarditis. Inflammation of all the structures in the heart, the outer covering, the muscular wall, the internal lining often resulting from rheumatic fever.

pancreas (*pahn'krih-uhss*). A large gland, six to eight inches long, lying in a horizontal position across the back wall of the abdominal cavity. The head of the gland on the right lies in contact with the first part of the small intestine. On the left, its tail is very close to the spleen. It produces a digestive juice that helps to break down proteins, fats, and carbohydrates that it empties through a duct into the small intestines. Within the substance of the gland are small islands of tissue known as the *Islets of Langerhans*. These areas produce insulin and expel it directly into the blood stream.

pancreatine (*paan'krih-uh-tihn*). A substance obtained from the fresh pancreas of the hog or ox that is commercially produced as a cream-colored powder and used for treatment of those cases in which there is an interference with digestion.

pancreatitis (*paan-krih-uh-tigh'tihss*). Inflammation of the pancreas that may be of very sudden onset with severe pain in the abdomen, vomiting, bloating, and pain on pressure in the abdomen; or may develop very slowly without any apparent symptoms until the function of the pancreas is seriously impaired.

pandemic. An epidemic over a very wide area.

pandiculation. The act of stretching and yawning on awakening.

panhysterectomy. The complete removal of the womb. Used loosely by many surgeons to mean removal of womb and the ovaries.

panniculitis (*paan-ih-kyuh-ligh'tihss*). Inflammation of the fat on the abdominal wall.

panniculus (*paa-nihk'yuh-luhss*). A layer of tissue. —*p. adiposus.* The layer of fat under the skin.

pannus. A growth of blood vessels in the transparent part of the eye often induced by the irritation of a disease, *trachoma*.

panophthalmitis (*paan-ahf-thaal-migh'tihss*). Inflammation of all the tissues of the eyeball.

pansinusitis. Inflammation of all the sinuses.

papilla (*puh-pihl'luh*). A small elevation, as a nipple; a pimple. —*duodenal p.* The elevation in the first part of the small intestine at the opening of the tube that brings in the bile. Also called *papilla of Vater.* —*gustatory p.* Elevations on the surface of the tongue that contain taste buds, seen readily on the back part of the tongue. —*lacrimal p.* A small, conelike elevation at the inner angle of the lower eyelid that has a visible hole and carries away tears. —*mammary p.* Breast nipple.

papilledema (*paap-ihl-ih-dee'muh*). Swelling of the nerve of sight where it enters the eyeball to become the retina.

papillitis. Inflammation of the head of the nerve of sight where it enters the eyeball. Also called *optic neuritis.*

papilloma. A tumor of skin, lining tissue, or glands, generally not dangerous, at times threatening to life.

papule (*paap'youl*). A small, solid elevation of the skin, varying in size from a pinpoint to a split-pea. Occurs in the course of a number of skin diseases.

papulopustular (*paap-you-loh-puhs'chuh-luhr*). Containing both papules and pimples with pus.

papulovesicular. Containing both papules and small blisters.

paracentesis (*paar-uh-sehn-tee'sihss*). Puncture. Especially used to mean the puncture of the wall of a body cavity by means of a hollow needle in order to draw out the fluid within it. —*abdominal p.* Puncture of the abdominal wall to remove fluid from the abdominal cavity, as in dropsy. —*p. of the bladder.* Puncture of the bladder wall to relieve the accumulating urine due to obstruction of the urinary flow. —*p. of the chest.* For relief of accumulating fluid in the space between the lungs and the chest wall. —*p. of the pericardium.* Puncture of the heart sac for relief of accumulating fluid that interferes with the action of the heart. —*p. of the tympanum.* Puncture of the eardrum to relieve accumulating matter in the middle ear.

paracusia (*paar-uh-kyou'zih-uh*). Any defection of the sense of hearing, as excessively acute hearing, ringing in the ears, difficulty in hearing, or difficulty in locating the direction of sound.

paraffinoma. A tumor mass of inflamed tissue or scar tissue resulting from the injection of paraffin into the tissue. Formerly paraffin was used under the tissues for reconstructing noses and in other plastic surgery.

paralysis. The inability of muscles to perform, caused by injury to the nerve or nerve cells. A slight loss of such ability is called *palsy*. —*acute ascending p.* A condition characterized by a limpness beginning in the muscles of the legs and spreading up the arms and other muscles of the body caused by a number of conditions; at times by infantile paralysis. Also called *Landry's p.* —*alcoholic p.* The chronic use of alcohol, particularly with insufficient food intake, may lead to injury of any one or a combination of nerves, and paralysis of the muscles they supply. —*arsenical p.* Numbness, tingling, and paralysis that comes on in late stages of arsenic poisoning. —*axillary p.* Paralysis of the muscle that lifts the arm from the side caused by a break or dislocation of the arm bone, or by pressure from a crutch. —*Bell's p.* Paralysis of the facial nerve with resulting paralysis of the muscles of expression in the face. —*cerebral p.* Paralysis due to an affection of cerebral centers. —*crutch p.* Paralysis of the muscles of the upper arm due to pressure from the head of the crutch. —*facial p.* Paralysis of the muscles of expression of the face. There are two types: the *central*, and the *peripheral*, or *Bell's palsy.* —*familial periodic p.* A hereditary condition of unknown cause, characterized by sudden attacks lasting a few hours to several days, of a paralysis of muscles in which the muscles are limp. —*general p. of the insane.* A form of syphilis of the brain characterized by tremors, seizures that resemble epilepsy, disturbances of speech, and mental changes. —*ginger p.* Paralysis of the legs and arms, chiefly due to the adulteration of liquor with a certain chemical. —*hysterical p.* Weakness or paralysis of the muscles without any evidence of physical disturbance. —*infantile p.* An infection of the nervous system caused by a virus characterized mainly by an abrupt onset with high fever and paralysis resulting in limpness and shrinking of muscle. Also called *acute anterior poliomyelitis.* —*jake p.* Paralysis of muscles due to involvement of nerve caused by drinking or eating Jamaica ginger. —*p. agitans.* A condition caused by the disintegration of part of the brain resulting in a slowing and weakness of movement and emotion, rigidity of the muscles, and a constant trembling. Also called *shaking palsy, Parkinsonism, Parkinson's disease.* —*progressive bulbar p.* A gradually increasing paralysis on both sides of the body, of the muscles of the face, throat, tongue, and at times of the voice box, due to disintegration of certain parts of the brain stem. —*pseudohypertrophic muscular p.* Loss or reduction in the power and movement of muscles accompanied by their seeming overdevelopment. —*Saturday night p.* Paralysis of the arm resulting from the compression of an arm nerve against the arm bone during sleep or when the arm is hung over the edge of a chair during intoxication. —*spinal p.* Paralysis due to an affection of spinal centers. —*Volkmann's p.* The paralysis of a hand due to great reduction or cutting off of its blood supply when splints or casts are applied too tightly to the forearm in the management of broken bones.

parametritis (*paar-uh-mih-trigh'tihss*). Inflammation of the tissue that surrounds and supports the womb.

parametrium. The tissue that surrounds and supports the womb.

paranasal. Situated near, or next to, the nose.

paranoia (*paar-uh-noy'uh*). A mental condition characterized by delusions of persecution, and hallucinations, usually of sound.

paraplegia (*paar-uh-plee'jih-uh*). Paralysis of the legs. —*alcoholic p.* Paralysis of the legs following alcoholic injury to nerves. —*ataxic p.* A condition that slowly increases in proportion characterized by continual spasm of the leg muscles, weakness, and inability to co-ordinate the movements of the leg. —*cerebral p.* Paralysis of both legs due to disturbance on both sides of the brain. —*congenital spastic p.* Paralysis of the legs with spasm of their muscles caused by a defect or injury in the brain existing from birth. Also called *Little's disease.* —*senile p.* Paralysis of the legs with spasm of their muscles as the result of hardening of the arteries of the spinal cord. —*spastic p.* Paralysis of the legs with spasm of the muscles seen in *multiple sclerosis* and other conditions in which the spinal cord is involved.

parapsychology. The study of extrasensory phenomena such as premonitions, mental telepathy, the knowledge of things to occur.

parasite. An organism that lives on or in another, known as the host, from which it obtains nourishment during part or all of its existence. Examples: the body louse; the bacteria that normally live in the mouth, nose, or throat; worms of the intestinal tract.

parasiticide (*paar-uh-siht'ih-sighd*). Destructive of parasites; any agent destroying parasites.

paraspadias. A condition in which the opening of the penis is on one side of the shaft.

parasympathetic. A part of the *autonomic nervous system,* which controls activity below the level of consciousness, as the secretion of glands, intestinal action, and heart action. The other component of this system is known as the *sympathetic nervous system.*

parateresiomania (*paar-uh-tehr-ih-zee-oh-may'nih-uh*). A compulsion for seeing new sights; a peeping mania.

parathyroid. One of four small endocrine glands that lie behind and in the outer corners of the thyroid gland. The hormone of these glands is concerned with the handling of phosphorus and calcium in the body. Removal of these glands results in a general spasm of the entire body called *tetany,* and death. Over- or underactivity of these glands has a definite effect upon bone formation or its dissolution.

paratonsillar. Near or around the tonsil.

paratyphoid. A generalized disease of man that comes on abruptly, and resembles typhoid fever but is less severe. Caused by paratyphoid bacteria, *Salmonella.*

parenchyma (*puh-rehn'kih-muh*). The productive part of an organ as distinguished from the supporting tissue. Examples: in the liver, the liver tissue excepting the fibrous tissue and its capsule that holds it together; in the lungs, the lung tissue, excepting the bronchial tubes and the fibrous tissue that divides it into the lobes.

parenteral (*puh-rehn′tuh-ruhl*). Outside of the intestine, as introduction of material into the body other than through the digestive tract or by mouth, an intravenous injection, a "hypo."

paresis (*puh-ree′sihss*). A minor paralysis; weakness of a part; incomplete loss of muscle power.

paresthesia. A tingling, burning, or crawling of the skin that occurs in certain involvements of nerves and the spinal cord.

pareunia (*puh-roo′nih-uh*). Sexual intercourse.

parietal (*puh-righ′uh-tuhl*). 1. (*adj.*) Situated on a wall, as the parietal layer of the tissue that lines the abdominal cavity and its contents. 2. (*n.*) The parietal bone, a bone forming part of the side and top of the skull.

parity. The state of being able to bear children.

paronychia (*paar-oh-nihk′ih-uh*). An inflammation with pus on the side of a nail.

parotid (*puh-raht′ihd*). Located near the ear, as the parotid gland, one of the glands that form saliva, commonly involved in mumps. 2. Relating to the parotid gland.

parotitis. Inflammation of the parotid gland, as in mumps.

parous. Having borne one or more children.

paroxysm (*paar′uhks-ihsm*). A sudden attack, a sudden increase in the intensity of symptoms, or a sudden reappearance of symptoms; a spasm or convulsion, as an attack of asthma.

parthenogenesis (*pahr-thuh-noh-jehn′uh-sihss*). A condition in which an organism develops from an egg that has not been penetrated by a male cell. Occurs chiefly in lower forms of life.

particulate. Made up of minute particles, as a spray of powder.

parturient. Giving birth, or being in labor.

parturition. The act of giving birth.

pasteurization. The process of heating milk, wine, or other fluids for 40 minutes to 60° or 70° centigrade in order to prevent fermentation and to destroy disease-producing germs.

past pointing. A test in which the patient is asked to point to a fixed object, alternately, with eyes open and shut. Example: the patient is asked to touch the finger of the examiner, first with eyes open, then with eyes shut; if there is a constant error with the eyes closed, a disturbance in the brain is probably present. Also called *Barany's pointing test.*

patella (*puh-tehl'luh*). The kneecap.

patency. The state of being open, as of blood vessels, ducts, and other hollow tubes or organs.

pathogen (*paath'uh-jehn*). A germ that is capable of producing disease.

pathogenic (*paath-uh-jehn'ihk*). Relating to the ability to produce disease.

pathognomonic (*paa-thahg-noh-mahn'ihk*). A special characteristic of a disease that distinguishes it from other diseases, as the presence of tuberculosis germs in the sputum is pathognomonic of respiratory tuberculosis.

pathology. The scientific specialty that deals with the nature of disease by studying its causes, its processes, its effects, and the alteration of the structure and performance of the tissue that it involves.

patulous (*paach'uh-luhs*). Open; expanded; often used in reference to the neck of the womb in a woman who has given birth to one or more children, as a *patulous cervix.*

pectoral. Referring to the chest, as the pectoral muscles that connect the arm with the chest.

pectus. The chest or breast. —*p. carinatum.* A narrow chest that projects in front in the region of the breast bone. Also called *chicken breast.* —*p. excavatum.* A deformity of the chest in which the breastbone is depressed toward the spine. Also called *funnel breast.*

pederasty (*pehd'uh-raas-tih*). Sexual intercourse through the anus.

pediatrics (*pee-dih-aat'rihks*). The specialty in medicine that deals with diseases in children from birth to age fourteen.

pediatrist (*pee-dih-aat'rihst*). A specialist in children's diseases. Also called *pediatrician*.

pedicular. Lousy, relating to lice.

pediculicide (*pih-dihk'yuh-lih-sighd*). Any agent that destroys lice.

pediculosis. A disease of the skin due to infestation with lice, characterized by intense itching and a rash. —*p. capitis.* Infestation of the scalp with lice, occurring chiefly in girls and women with long hair. —*p. corporis.* Infestation of the body skin with lice. If the condition has been present for a long time, the constant scratching causes the skin to thicken and develop spots of color. Also called *Vagabond's disease.* —*p. pubis.* Infestation of the hair in the pubic region with lice; may spread over the body and involve the armpit, the eyebrows, and the eyelashes. Called, in the vernacular, "crabs."

Pediculus. The general name for lice, some of which cause inflammation of the skin and transmit diseases, as trench fever. —*p. humanus variety capitis.* The head louse. —*p. humanus variety corporis.* The body louse, an important carrier of disease.

pelada (*pih-lahd'uh*). Patchy baldness of the scalp.

pelage (*pehl'ihj*). The hairy covering of the body.

pellagra (*puh-laa'gruh*). A disease caused by a deficiency in food intake, occurring particularly in southern U. S., Italy, southern France, and Spain, and other areas. Pellagra is characterized by loss of strength, digestive disturbances, pain up and down the spine, and a redness, drying, and peeling of the skin. In the very serious cases, nervous manifestations may arise, as spasms, paralysis, and mental deficiency. A good diet with a great deal of *niacin*, one of the vitamin-B complex, cures the condition unless serious changes in the nervous system have already taken place.

pellicle. 1. A thin tissue. 2. A film or scum on the surface of a liquid, as the film that develops on the surface of heated milk.

pelvimeter (*pehl-vihm'ih-tuhr*). An instrument for measuring the various dimensions of the bony pelvic girdle used to determine the adequacy of the passageway for the developing infant in pregnant women. Definite narrowing of the pelvic passage may be an indication for a Caesarian delivery.

pelvis. 1. A basin or basin-shaped cavity. 2. The structure formed by the bones into which the head of the thigh bone and the very lower end of the spine fit. 3. The cavity that is bounded by this bony structure containing in the female the rectum, anus, womb, urinary bladder, Fallopian tubes, ovaries, and parts of the tubes (the ureters) that lead from the kidney to the bladder; in the male, all of these structures except the ovaries, Fallopian tubes, and womb. —*contracted p.* A pelvis with reduced major dimensions interfering with childbirth. —*funnel p.* A deformity in the pelvis with normal outer measurements and a greatly contracted outlet through which the fetus passes in childbirth, and is much like a funnel, wide at the top and narrow at the bottom. —*justo-major p.* A pelvis generally enlarged. —*justo-minor p.* A pelvis generally smaller than normal. —*renal p.* A large, funnel-shaped part of the kidney, the collecting area for urine that narrows down and becomes the ureter, or the tube that leads to the bladder.

pemphigus (*pehm'fih-guhss*). A disease of the skin that is characterized by crops of large blisters. —*p. acutis.* A disease that appears frequently in butchers or trappers, caused by a germ derived from dead or living animals. A serious condition in which the skin of the entire body is affected, and the patient is extremely sick for several weeks; often results in death. —*p. vulgaris.* A condition of long duration, characterized by crop after crop of blisters that leave colored spots in the skin after they heal.

pendulous (*pehn'juh-luhss*). Loosely hanging down, as pendulous breasts.

penis. The male organ of sexual intercourse, composed of three cylinders arranged in triangular form, the top cylinder lying upon the two bottom cylinders that are adjacent to each other. The top cylinder, the *corpus spongiosum*, encloses the passageway of the penis, the urethra, through which urine and semen traverse. The two bottom cylinders, the *corpora cavernosa*, consist of elastic tissue with large empty spaces that fill with blood and cause erection of the penis. —*p. captivus*. A penis held in the vagina during intercourse by the sharp spasm of the female muscles.

percussion. The act of tapping the surface of the body with the finger or a small hammer in order to elicit sound or vibrations that are of use in making a diagnosis. Different pitches of sound indicate the condition of the organs or the cavity being percussed.

perianal (*pehr-ih-ay'nuhl*). Located, or occurring, around the anus.

periarteritis (*pehr-ih-ahr-tuh-righ'tihss*). Inflammation of the outer coat of an artery and of the tissues surrounding the artery. —*p. nodosa*. A severe inflammation of all the layers of the walls of the small arteries with the formation of small lumps of inflammation along the outer walls. May occur in any of the small arteries throughout the body and symptoms may refer to any of the organs or systems of the body, as brain, stomach and intestinal, kidney, and liver symptoms. Frequently fatal and thought to be allergic.

periarticular. Surrounding a joint.

pericardiectomy. Surgical removal of part of the heart sac. Performed where there is shrinkage of the heart sac with compression of the heart, or where adhesions form between the heart sac and the chest wall, or the heart sac and the heart muscle.

pericarditis. Inflammation of the sac surrounding the heart. Symptoms are mild fever, pain and tenderness in the region of the heart, difficulty in breathing, cough, and rapid pulse. Liquid may accumulate in the heart sac causing an increase in symptoms and greater difficulty for the heart to beat. Pericarditis results from rheumatic fever, blood poisoning, tuberculosis, kidney disease, an infection in the parts surrounding the heart, and at times cancer of the heart sac. Pericarditis is a serious condition and may leave the individual a heart cripple.

pericardium. The sac that envelops the heart and ordinarily contains about a whiskey-jigger of clear liquid.

perimetrium. The covering tissue of the womb.

perineorrhaphy (*pehr-ih-nee-awr'ruh-fih*). The surgical sewing of the tissue between the vagina and the anus, usually for the repair of a tear that occurs during childbirth.

perineotomy. A surgical stabbing through the tissue between the vagina or the upper end of the scrotum and the anus.

perinephric. Located or occurring about the kidneys, as a perinephric abscess.

perineum (*pehr-ih-nee'uhm*). The region between the anus and the scrotum in the male; between the anus and the vaginal opening in the female.

periodicity. Recurrence at regular intervals, as of menstruation.

period of gestation. The time from conception until childbirth, approximately 280 days in humans. To obtain the approximate date of confinement count back three months from the first day of the last period and add seven days.

perionychia (*pehr-ih-oh-nihk'ih-uh*). Inflammation around the finger or toenail.

periosteum (*pehr-ih-ahss'tih-uhm*). A thin tough tissue that covers the surface of bones, except at the points where tendons and ligaments attach and where the bone makes up part of a joint.

periostitis. Inflammation of the tissue covering the surface of bone, caused by infection or injury, of sudden or slow onset and short or long duration.

peristalsis. A wave of alternate contraction and relaxation that travels the length of the intestine from the stomach, forcing its contents toward its opening.

peritoneoscope. A hollow instrument, much like a long slender telescope, through which instruments are passed, and the abdominal cavity into which it is introduced is visualized.

peritoneum (*pehr-ih-tuh-nee'uhm*). The thin lining tissue that covers the walls of, and the organs in, the abdominal cavity.

peritonitis (*pehr-ih-tuh-nigh'tihss*). Inflammation of the tissue lining the organs and walls of the abdominal cavity. Peritonitis may be of severe, sudden onset, accompanied by pain in the abdomen, tenderness to touch, vomiting, fever, and inability to evacuate the bowels due to infection or irritation. It may·be of slow onset and long duration as a result of such diseases as tuberculosis and mold infections. Most commonly spread by infection from a diseased organ, the rupture of an organ, a gathering abscess, or injury.

peritonsillar. Around the tonsil.

permeability. The property of tissues that permits the passage of fluid through them. *—capillary p.* The property of capillaries that permits passage through their walls of various elements from the blood into the surrounding tissues, and from the surrounding tissues into the blood.

pernicious. Extremely severe. Unusually destructive. Possibly fatal, as pernicious anemia, pernicious vomiting of pregnancy.

per os (*puhr ahss'*). By mouth, as in administration of medicine; a tablet, elixir, capsule is given *per os* in contradistinction to an injection, inhalation, ointment, or medicine via the rectum.

personality. The sum total of characteristics and ways of behavior of an individual as they seem to others. Regarded as the result of the interplay between the forces of society and the instincts with which the individual is born. *—alternating p.* One in which the individual may live alternately as two different persons, also called *dual personality*, e.g., a Dr. Jekyll and Mr. Hyde. *—cycloid p.* One characterized by periods of markedly increased mental and physical activity, alternating with others of inactivity or depression. —*multiple p.* Similar to *alternating p.* except that more than two personalities may be assumed by the individual, often a symptom of schizophrenia. —*psychopathic p.* A personality that is characterized by lack of awareness of moral responsibility, defects in judgment, emotional immaturity, impulsive behavior without consideration for others, and general behavior that indicates not having learned much from past experience. The psychopathic personality is an individual who will commit a crime of any degree without feeling remorse or being aware of his act as an offense against society.

pes (*pehs*). A foot, or footlike structure. —*p. contortis.* Clubfoot. —*p. planus.* Flatfoot.

pessary (*pehs'suh-rih*). An appliance of varied form placed in the vagina either to correct a bad position of the womb or to prevent conception.

petechia (*pih-tee'kih-uh*). A tiny pinpoint or pinhead spot of bleeding in the skin or lining tissues or within an organ.

petrositis (*piht-roh-sigh'tihss*). Inflammation of part of the temple bone that extends into the skull cavity, usually the result of an extension of infection from a mastoid or the middle ear.

phagocyte (*faag-oh-sight*). The general name for types of cells that have the property of engulfing and digesting foreign particles or other cells harmful to the body. One of the middle echelon defense mechanisms of the body.

phalanx. One of the bones of the fingers or toes.

phallus. The penis.

pharmacopeia (*fahr-muh-koh-pee'uh*). A standard book of formulas and methods of preparations of drugs recognized as a standard. Examples: the U. S. or British pharmacopeia. The U. S. pharmacopeia is brought up to date every five years under the supervision of a national committee.

pharyngectomy (*faar-ihn-jehk'tuh-mih*). The surgical removal of part of the throat.

pharyngitis. Inflammation of the throat caused by infection or irritation. Pharyngitis may be of sudden onset and marked severity characterized by pain on swallowing, dryness, phlegm, and congestion of the lining tissue of the throat; or it may come on gradually and remain for a long period as the end result of the more severe form just mentioned, or of constant irritation.

pharyngoscope. An instrument for examining the throat.

pharynx. A tube whose wall is made of muscle lined by mucous membrane situated behind the nose, mouth, and voice box, and extending from the base of the skull down to a level just above the shoulders. Below, it becomes continuous with the gullet or esophagus. The upper part of the pharynx communicates with the nose through the two hind openings of the nose, known as the *naso-pharynx*. The middle section of the pharynx communicates with the mouth, the *oro-pharynx*. Below the level of the mouth the pharynx is known as the *laryngo-pharynx*, lying behind the voice box. There are two openings into the pharynx just behind the tonsils that represent the outlets of the *auditory tubes* leading into the middle ear.

philtrum. The shallow vertical trough on the upper lip below the nose.

phimosis (*figh-moh'sihss*). A lengthening of the foreskin and narrowing of its opening so that it cannot be pulled back over the tip of the penis. Usually requires circumcision.

phlebitis. Inflammation of a vein, usually the result of extension of infection from near-by tissues, that leads to formation of a clot within the vein (*thrombophlebitis*). The clot may break into many pieces and be carried as particles of infection to various parts of the body, causing trouble there. When not due to infection (*plastic, proliferative, adhesive phlebitis*), the vein may become entirely closed off. Symptoms are swelling of the involved parts, as a leg; pain; and redness along the vein with the vein taking on the appearance of a hard, tender cord.

phlebolith (*flehb'oh-lihth*). A small, hard mass, similar to a stone, at times found in a vein. Produced by the laying down of calcium salts in a clot.

phlebosclerosis. The hardening of a vein similar to the hardening of arteries, often the result of long-standing inflammation.

phlebothrombosis. The formation of a clot in a vein.

Phlebotomus (*fleh-baht'uh-muhss*). The general name of various kinds of bloodsucking sandflies that are responsible for the transmission of a number of diseases to man.

phlebotomy (*fleh-baht'uh-mih*). Bloodletting from a vein. Used at times in high blood pressure. Examples: obtaining blood from blood donors; drawing blood from a vein for various laboratory tests.

phlegm (*flehm*). A stringy mucus produced by the lining tissue of the upper air passages.

phlegmatic (*flehg-maat'ihk*). Of a sluggish, disinterested character.

phlegmon (*flehg'mahn*). Pus-forming inflammation of a part, particularly of fibrous tissue.

phlyctenule (*flihk-tehn'yuhl*). A tiny blister, commonly part of a general inflammation of the eyeball or lids.

phobia. An obsessive fear that accompanies emotional or mental disorders, as the fear of open spaces, height, crowds.

phonocardiography. The procedure by which the sounds of the heart are recorded on paper.

photodynia (*foh-toh-dihn'ih-uh*). Pain in the eyes from exposure to great intensity of light.

photomicrograph. A photograph of a microscopic object, made with a camera attached to a microscope. Used as a permanent record of microscopic changes in tissues, and in the study of microscopic life.

photophobia. Eye pain on exposure to light, or a morbid fear of light. A mild form of photodynia.

photophthalmia (*foh-tahf-thaal'mih-uh*). Inflammation of the eyes from exposure to the unusually strong light of a welder's arc or sunlight on snow.

photosensitization. An excessive sensitivity of the skin to sunlight or to ultraviolet light, often resulting in inflammation of the skin with large hives or other eruption. Occurs independently or as part of the condition known as *lupus erythematosis.*

phrenic (*frehn'ihk*). 1. Relating to the diaphragm, as the phrenic nerve, the nerve of the diaphragm. 2. Relating to the mind.

phrenicectomy (*frehn-ih-sehk'tuh-mih*). The surgical removal of a part of or the entire phrenic nerve. This operation is used in the treatment of tuberculosis of the lung when it is necessary to give the lung a measure of rest. By interrupting the phrenic nerve, one side of the diaphragm is paralyzed, resulting in much less movement of the lung on that side.

phrenicotomy. A cutting across of the phrenic nerve in its course through the neck. The incision is made in the neck above the middle of the collarbone. This operation is performed for the same purpose as a phrenicectomy.

phrenicotripsy (*frehn-ih-koh-trihp'sih*). An operation for immobilization of the lung by crushing the phrenic nerve with a metal forceps.

phrenoplegia (*frehn-oh-plee'jih-uh*). Paralysis of the diaphragm.

phthisiology (*tihz-ih-ahl'uh-jih*). The science or study of tuberculosis.

phthisis (*thigh'sihss*). An archaic term for tuberculosis, particularly of the lung; or for any disease, especially of the lungs, that results in wasting away and loss of strength.

phylaxis. The body's action in defending itself against infection; any treatment that aids the body in this defense action, as giving tetanus antitoxin to a patient with lockjaw.

physiology. The science that deals with the functions of living organisms, as distinguished from anatomy, which deals with the structure of organs and parts. Anatomy is concerned with what organs and parts are and how they are built; physiology with what they do and how they do it.

phytosis. Any disease caused by vegetable parasites, or the production of disease by vegetable parasites, or the presence of vegetable parasites. Example: infection with yeast.

phytotoxin. A toxin or poison produced by a plant, as *ricin* produced by the castor bean.

pia mater (*pigh'uh may'tuhr*). The innermost covering of the brain and spinal cord composed of many blood vessels held together by a fine mesh of thin tissue.

pica (*pigh'kuh*). A craving for strange foods during pregnancy; a craving for and eating of strange things as dirt, coal, cinders, occurring very frequently in children, and at times late in life.

pile. A hemorrhoid. An enlarged vein of the anus engorged with blood. —*blind p.* One without bleeding. —*external p.* One that is below the muscle that closes and opens the anus. —*internal p.* One that is above this muscle.

pilomotor (*pigh-loh-moh'tuhr*). Inducing the movement of the hair, as the nerve that supplies the muscles at the base of the hair. These nerves are responsible for the pimply appearance of skin on exposure to cold or to an emotional reaction, known as "gooseflesh."

pilonidal (*pigh-loh-nigh'duhl*). The name given a cyst that contains hairs, not infrequently found at the base of the spine. May cause trouble by seepage, becoming infected and producing pain. Usually requires complete removal by surgery.

pineal gland (*pigh'nih-uhl*). A small, cone-shaped gland, a fraction of an inch long, that lies at the base of the brain near the pituitary gland. The purpose it serves is not entirely clear, but it is known to be related to sexual precocity in male children.

pinkeye. A contagious inflammation of the eye with the production of matter and a very definite reddening of the whites of the eyes. Also called *Koch-Weeks conjunctivitis*.

pipette. A glass tube marked off in various measurements used for transferring exact quantities of liquid. The amount of fluid desired is sucked into the tube and kept in place by covering the upper opening with the thumb. When transferred to the receiving container, release of thumb forces the fluid out.

pisiform (*pigh'sih-fawrm*). A small, pea-shaped bone on the inner and front part of the wrist.

pituitary. A most important gland of internal secretion that lies in the mid-part of the skull at the base of the brain in a bony depression known as the *Turkish Saddle*. Directly in front of the gland, the nerves of sight cross to enter the eyeballs and become the retina. This gland produces many hormones. From the front part of the gland, the *anterior lobe*, come hormones regulating the growth of all the tissues in the body, controlling the growth and production of the thyroid gland, the outer shell of the adrenal, the testes, the ovaries, the parathyroid gland, and the secretion of milk. The back part, or the *posterior lobe* of the gland, produces hormones that regulate blood pressure, the workability of the muscles not under the control of the will, and the working of the kidneys. Many injectable hormones are made from the pituitary glands of cattle, sheep, and hogs, among them ACTH.

pityriasis (*piht-ih-righ'uh-sihss*). A fine, branlike shedding of skin that occurs in a number of conditions. —*p. rosea.* A skin disease of unknown cause, limited usually to the trunk, coming on suddenly, and disappearing ordinarily in from four to six weeks. The eruption is one of pale-red patches with beige-colored centers. —*p. rubra.* An inflammatory disease of the skin that ordinarily involves the entire body. The skin is deep red and covered with gray or white scales. It may last months or years and is often fatal. —*p. versicolor.* A skin disease involving mostly the trunk with large yellow-brown, scaling spots, due to a fungus.

placebo (*pluh-see'boh*). A medicine that has no effect, but that is given to the patient to satisfy his need for a medicine or in an attempt to determine whether or not relief by previous medication was physical or emotional. Examples: sugar pills, bread crumb pills, capsules containing inert materials.

placenta. The organ that develops on the wall of the womb about the third month after conception, and to which the developing infant is attached by means of the umbilical cord. The placenta is formed partially from the lining tissue of the womb and partially from the sac that surrounds the developing infant. Through the placenta, that has many finger-like projections growing into the wall of the womb, food and other necessary elements are brought to the developing infant and waste products from the infant are channeled out into the mother's blood stream. There is no direct connection between the blood of the mother and the blood of the infant. The two blood streams are separated by the very thin walls of the placental projections. After childbirth the placenta is expelled. Ordinarily, the placenta weighs about one pound, is about one inch thick, and about 7 inches in diameter. It is popularly called the afterbirth. —*adherent p.* One that does not separate from the wall of the womb after childbirth but must be helped out by the obstetrician. —*p. previa.* One that is implanted very low in the womb near or about the opening, often producing serious bleeding during labor and episodes of bleeding before completion of the pregnancy.

plague. 1. Any serious, contagious, epidemic disease. 2. A specific condition, the *bubonic plague*, that is particularly prevalent in eastern Asia and earlier occurred in epidemics in Europe and Asia Minor. Bubonic plague is a disease of sudden onset with high fever, inflammation of the lymph vessels, formation of large swellings of the lymph glands, pinpoint bleeding under the skin, in the lining tissues, and within various organs, severe bleeding externally, development of pneumonia, and often death. The germ that causes plague is *Pasteurella pestis*, transmitted by fleas from rats to man. In the fourteenth century this condition was called the

Black Plague because of the great proportion of hemorrhages that occurred.

plantar. Relating to the sole of the foot.

plantaris. A very small muscle that, with the gastrocnemius and soleus, makes up the calf of the leg.

plantar wart. A type of wart that appears on the bottom of the foot and becomes very painful. Because of pressure the wart cannot grow out from the surface. Also called *verruca plantaris.*

plasma. The blood without its cells; the liquid part of the blood.

Plasmodium. A type of single-celled, microscopic animal that produces malaria. There are four types: *p. falciparum*, causing serious *tertian malaria*; *p. vivax*, causing *tertian malaria* of the mild variety; *p. malariae*, causing *quartan malaria*; *p. ovale*, causing *tertian malaria*. If different species of plasmodium circulate in the blood they may cause daily recurring attacks of fever, *i.e., quotidian malaria.*

plastic. 1. Concerned with repairing defects or malformations, restoring lost parts, building up tissues, as plastic surgery. 2. The quality of being moldable. 3. Any material that can be molded.

platelet (*playt'liht*). A small, colorless disc present in the blood stream; about 250,000 to 500,000 per cubic millimeter of blood; important in clotting of blood. Also called *thrombocyte.*

platysma (*plaa-tihz'muh*). A thin, flat, wide muscle immediately under the skin of the neck that extends from the jaw bone to the collar bone.

pleasure principle. The principle governing the striving of the organism for satisfaction of its drives and fulfillment of its wishes. The pleasure principle is the mechanism characteristic of the id, as opposed to the control and inhibition of drives and wishes by the superego. *See also* ID and SUPEREGO.

pledget (*plehj'eht*). A flattened, small piece of cotton or gauze, soaked in alcohol or other antiseptic, often used to cover an area of skin.

pleura (*ploor'uh*). The thin tissue that covers the lungs and lines the interior walls of the chest cavity.

pleurisy (*ploo'ruh-sih*). Inflammation of the pleura, also called pleuritis. —*acute p.* A condition that comes on suddenly with fever and pain on breathing or coughing or any other movement that jars the chest, and results from blood poisoning, pneumonia, or inflammation of organs in the chest other than the lungs. —*adhesive p.* A condition in which the pleura lining the chest wall adheres to the pleura covering the lungs. —*chronic p.* A type that develops slowly with adhesions between the pleura covering the lung and the pleura lining the chest wall; often seen in tuberculosis. —*diaphragmatic p.* Inflammation of the pleura covering the upper surface of the diaphragm. —*purulent p.* Inflammation of the pleura with formation of pus. Also called *empyema, pyothorax.*

pleurodynia (*ploo-ruh-dihn'ih-uh*). A sharp pain in the muscles between the ribs. —*epidemic p.* A disease of sudden onset with fever, pain in the chest and just below the breastbone and along the sides of the spine. Also called *devil's grip, Bornholm's disease.*

plexus. A meshwork; applied to interlacing nerves, blood vessels, or lymph vessels.

pneumoencephalography (*nyou-moh-ehn-sehf-uh-lohg'ruh-fih*). Within the brain there are large, sac-like spaces known as *ventricles*, filled with a fluid called the *cerebrospinal fluid.* In order to X-ray the brain and to determine the presence of disease here, it is necessary to introduce into these ventricles a material that will show up on X-ray. By removing some of the spinal fluid from low in the spinal canal and replacing it with air, the air rises into the ventricle system and when an X-ray is taken, the system is outlined on the X-ray film. In this manner, obstruction and compression of the ventricle system can be determined.

pneumonectomy. The surgical removal of an entire lung.
pneumonia. Inflammation of the lung. Also called pneumonitis. —*aspiration p.* Caused by inhalation of fluid or food into the lungs, a condition that often occurs when a general anesthetic is given. —*hypostatic p.* Infection of the lower parts of the lungs due to the individual remaining in one position for too long a time; usually seen in aged people. —*lipid p.* Resulting from the inhalation of oily substances such as nose drops, cod liver oil, oily vitamin preparations, and mineral oils into the passageways of the lung. Particularly seen in children and in adults whose cough reflex is impaired. —*lobar p.* A pneumonia that comes on suddenly with fever due to infection with a particular type of germ, the *pneumococcus*. There is rapid breathing, cough with a rusty-colored expectoration, pain, and general sickness. After about a week the fever drops within a 24-hour period. The lungs are divided into five parts, three on the right, and two on the left. These parts are known as lobes. In lobar pneumonia, one or more lobes of the lung are involved. Since the advent of penicillin and the sulfa drugs, this condition is a rarity. At one time it was responsible for many deaths. —*virus p.* A type of pneumonia caused by one of a number of viruses characterized by fever, cough, general weakness, and a prolonged course. It usually disappears and does not respond to the sulfa drugs or to the antibiotics. Here the lungs are not involved by lobes but rather in patches throughout. Also called *primary atypical p.*
pneumonoconiosis (*nyou-moh-noh-koh-nih-oh'sihss*). An inflammation of the lungs coming on slowly, lasting for a long time, and caused by the inhalation of various mineral dusts. Examples are *silicosis*, from inhalation of dust containing *silica*, as in quarry workers, stonecutters, and occasionally in sculptors; *asbestosis*, from dust of asbestos; *anthracosis*, from carbon dust in coal miners; *siderosis*, from iron dust; and many others.
pneumothorax. The presence of gas or air in the space be-

tween the lung and the chest wall, the result of wounds that perforate the chest; the rupture of an abscess or a cavity close to the surface of the lung; often caused by tuberculosis. —*artificial p.* The intentional introduction of air or gas into the space between the lungs and the chest wall in order to collapse the lung and put it to rest, at the same time closing any cavities within the lung. Used commonly in the treatment of tuberculosis of the lung. —*spontaneous p.* Nonintentional pneumothorax.

podagra (*poh-daag'ruh*). Gout, particularly of the large toe, or the joints of the foot.

podiatrist (*poh-digh'uh-trihst*). A specialist (usually not a physician) in the treatment of diseases of the feet. Also called *chiropodist*.

point. A minute spot or area. —*McBurney's p.* A point, halfway between the navel and the sharp prominent tip of bone on the upper front part of the hip, painful to the touch in acute appendicitis.

poison. A substance that, on entering the blood, ends life or seriously damages one or more of the body organs.

poisoning. The state produced by a poison. —*food p.* A general term referring to poisoning due to foods contaminated by bacterial poisons, or by living bacteria themselves; or to foods that in themselves are poisonous, as certain mushrooms; or to foods contaminated by chemicals; or to foods that cause a serious allergic reaction in the patient.

poison ivy. A vine that causes a severe irritation of the skin due to an oily substance within it called *urushiol.*

poison oak. A shrub with leaves that resemble oak leaves and contain an irritating substance producing an inflammation of the skin similar to poison ivy.

poison sumac. A shrub that contains an oil poisonous to the touch, producing a condition resembling *poison ivy dermatitis.*

poliomyelitis. Inflammation of the gray matter of the spinal cord. —*acute anterior p.* An inflammation of the gray matter of the spinal cord, coming on abruptly with fever, stomach and intestinal complaints, and pain in the affected muscles. Paralysis is usually greatest in the beginning. A certain amount of improvement almost always takes place later. Due to the muscle involvement, deformities may occur in later life. The disease appears in epidemic flare-ups. Many patients do not go on to paralysis, and it is believed that many others have very mild forms of the disease, not recognizable, from which they derive a life-long immunity. Also called *epidemic paralysis, acute wasting paralysis, infantile paralysis*.

pollen. The male sex cells of plants.

pollenosis. Allergy to pollen that shows itself in symptoms, as hay fever, asthma, dermatitis, conjunctivitis.

pollex. The thumb.

pollution. 1. Defiling or making impure, as pollution of water. 2. Discharge of semen without sexual intercourse. Also called *nocturnal emission*.

polyarthritis. Inflammation of many joints. Used loosely to mean acute rheumatic fever.

polycythemia (*pahl-ih-sigh-thee'mih-uh*). A condition in which the number of red blood cells is increased considerably above normal. —*primary p.* A rare condition in which the increase in the red cells is due to an overworking of the bone marrow that forms them without any known cause. This condition is manifested by a reddish-blue complexion; disturbance of the nervous system, the stomach, and intestines; nosebleeds; and an unusual enlargement of the spleen. The outlook for life is not good. One of the frequent complications is massing of the red blood cells into large particles because of their excess number and the blocking of vital blood vessels. —*secondary p.* An increase in the red blood cells frequently produced by a long-standing heart condition. Where the heart is inefficient in circulating the blood, the body attempts to compensate for this by increasing the number of red blood cells so that oxygen in sufficient amount can be taken up and carbon dioxide given off.

polydypsia. Excessive thirst.

polyhydramnios. An excessive production of fluid within the sac containing the developing infant.

polyp. A gourdlike tumor growing from lining tissues of hollow organs, such as of the nose, the stomach, the intestines, the womb, the bladder. —*nasal p.* A gourdlike or flattened mass projecting from the tissue lining the nose. It may be multiple and small or single and large, at times protruding from the nose, and almost always allergic in nature. Except for mechanical blockage of the nose, it is not serious.

polyphagia (*pahl-ih-fay'jih-uh*). Excessive eating. Also called *bulimia*.

polyuria. Passage of an excessive amount of urine.

pons. 1. A bridge of tissue that connects two parts of an organ. 2. A specific part at the base of the brain in which many important pathways of nervous fibers pass from the gray matter to the cerebellum, that part of the brain concerned with co-ordination and balance.

popliteal (*pahp-lih-tee'uhl*). Relating to the area at the back of the leg, and in the bend of the knee. Also called the *ham*.

port wine mark. A kind of mole, purple or violet in color, only slightly raised above the skin, usually seen on the face. A type of birthmark.

position. An attitude, posture. —*Fowler's p.* The position of a patient in bed with the head raised 18 to 20 inches above the feet. This position is accomplished by a back rest or by blocks under the head of the bed. —*knee-chest p.* The position of the patient resting on the knees and chest, used as an exercise after childbirth, or for examination and treatment. —*Sims's p.* The patient on the left side, the left arm along the back, the right knee and thigh drawn up and the chest bent forward, used by some obstetricians for delivery. —*Trendelenburg's p.* The position of a patient lying on a table, the foot of which is tilted up 45°, the legs and feet of the patient hanging over the elevated end.

postcoital (*pohst-koh'ih-tuhl*). After sexual intercourse.

posterior. Located behind or at the back of a part.

posthumous (*pahs'choo-muhss*). Occurring after death.

post-mortem. An examination of a body after death, an autopsy.

postnasal. Located behind the nose.

postnatal. Immediately after birth.

postoperative. Occurring after an operation, as a rupture, infection.

postpartum. Following on childbirth, as *postpartum psychosis*.

postprandial. After a meal.

potency. The power of the male to perform the sex act.

preclinical. 1. Before the time when symptoms and signs appear, as the period between infection with germs and the appearance of symptoms.

pregnancy. Bearing a child. Also called gestation. —*abdominal p.* At times the egg cell that has been penetrated by the sperm does not settle into the womb wall, but finds its way back through one of the tubes and drops into the abdominal cavity. The development of the infant will go on for a time in this unusual location. Complete development never occurs. —*phantom p.* Many or all of the symptoms of pregnancy, usually due to a type of hysteria. Also called *pseudocyesis.* —*tubal p.* The development of the fertilized egg cell within one of the tubes; always requires surgery.

prenatal. Occurring before birth.

prepatellar (*pree-puh-tehl'luhr*). Located in front of the kneecap.

prepuce (*pree'pyouss*). The foreskin, either of the penis or of the clitoris.

presbyopia (*prehz-bih-oh'pih-uh*). A defection of vision that comes on with age caused by a loss of the elastic quality of the lens that becomes fixed in an elongated form. As a result, near objects are not seen clearly. This is why many older people hold printed matter at arm's length for reading.

presentation. The part of the developing infant that is felt by the examining finger through the opening of the neck of the womb when ready to be delivered. There are many types: *breech p.*, where the buttocks or the feet are present at the opening; *brow p.*, where the brow is present; *cephalic p.*, where any part of the head is present; *face p.*, where the face with the chin foremost presents; *transverse p.*, where the developing infant lies across the width of the womb and the presenting part may be the abdomen, back, and shoulder; *vertex p.*, where the back of the head presents first, the most usual type.

presystolic. Systole commonly refers to the period when the large chambers of the heart, the ventricles, are squeezing out blood into the general circulation. In the normal rhythm of the heart there is a period of pause immediately before this. Presystolic refers to this period and especially to the time immediately before the first heart sound.

priapism (*prigh'uh-pihsm*). The continued and persistent erection of the penis ordinarily not accompanied by sexual desire; may be extremely painful and occurs not infrequently as a symptom in leukemia, a serious blood disease.

primigravida (*prigh-mih-graav'ih-duh*). A woman pregnant for the first time.

primipara (*prigh-mihp'uh-ruh*). A woman giving birth to her first child.

probe. A thin, flexible rod, often of metal, made for exploring or increasing the size of a natural channel or one caused by disease.

process. An outgrowth of a part, such as an extension of bone, or the prolongation of parts of a cell.

proctitis. Inflammation of the rectum or anus.

proctoclysis (*prahk-toh-kligh'sihss*). The slow introduction of a liquid into the rectum, usually as a means of feeding, supplying with fluid, or with medication.

proctology. The study of the rectum, its structure, actions, and diseases.

proctoscopy (*prahk-tahs'kuh-pih*). The visual inspection of the rectum with the aid of a special instrument.

prodrome. The early symptoms of a disease that appear before the characteristic symptoms. Examples: the general weakness and lack of interest that may occur for a day or two before the onset of an infectious disease; the unusual sense of smell or general achiness that people with migraine develop before the headache itself comes on. A premonitory symptom of a disease.

progeria (*proh-jee'rih-uh*). Senility appearing before its time in which characteristics of infantilism are displayed. Also called *Hutchinson-Gilford disease*.

prognathism (*prahg'nuh-thism*). The state of having projecting jaws.

prognosis. A prediction of how a disease will progress from point of view of time, termination, and course, based on all the information the physician has both in regard to the patient himself and the disease in general.

projection. The process of attributing to other persons or things the ideas or impulses that are one's own. Underlying this process is the implication that the ideas or impulses so attributed to others are undesirable in oneself. The mechanism behind this process is an unconscious one of which the individual is not aware. A common example is blaming another for one's own mistakes. Certain psychotics with homosexual urges project these urges upon other persons. In directing their attacks against these persons they actually struggle against their own urges, which now seem to them to have an origin outside of themselves.

prolapse. The sinking down or the falling of a part. —*frank p.* The downward falling of the womb through the vaginal canal, carrying with it the walls of the vagina so that they hang outside the vaginal opening.

prominence. A projection or elevation especially on a bone. —*laryngeal p.* A projection on the major section of gristle that makes up the front of the voice box. Also called *Adam's apple*.

pronate. To turn the forearm so that the palm of the hand is down or toward the back.

prone. Lying with face downward.

prophylaxis. The prevention of disease, or the measures used to prevent the spread or development of disease, as small pox vaccination, shots against diphtheria and tetanus given to children.

proprietary (*pruh-prigh'uh-tuhr-ih*). Any medicine used in the treatment of disease that is patented, copyrighted, or that employs any other measure against use of this medicine by the same name. Example: Adrenalin, a Parke-Davis name for *epinephrin*. A proprietary medicine is distinct from a patent medicine, the former being sold only on prescription and advertised only to the medical profession, whereas the latter is sold without prescription to the general public.

prostate (*prahs'tayt*). A gland in the male that is situated around the neck and exit of the urinary bladder and through which runs the beginning of the urethra (the passageway for urine from the bladder through the penis and out). The prostate consists of two large lobes connected by a small middle lobe, and is composed of muscular and glandular tissue. One of its major functions is to secrete *prostatic fluid*, that unites with the semen and gives it its liquid quality. Often, in later life, it becomes enlarged, obstructing the passage of urine.

prostatectomy. The surgical removal of all or part of the prostate. —*perineal p.* The removal of the prostate through an incision in the perineum, the space between the scrotum and the anus. —*suprapubic p.* The surgical removal of the prostate through an incision in the abdominal wall below the navel and through the bladder. —*transurethral p.* The removal of the middle lobe of the prostate by the use of an instrument that is inserted into the urethra (the passageway through the penis). Electrical current is the method of removal. Also called *transurethral resection*.

prostatitis (*prahs-tuh-tigh'tihss*). Inflammation of the prostate gland.

prosthesis. The making and fitting of an artificial substitute for a missing part, such as a false leg, hand, eye, teeth.

prostration. Extreme exhaustion. Refers to such a state due to disease or injury.

protein. A particular type of complex organic substance found in plants and animals, characteristic of living matter. Characterized by the presence of nitrogen in its molecule. —*plasma proteins*. The general name for the three kinds of protein present in the fluid part of the blood: *fibrinogen*, that plays a part in the clotting of blood; *globulins*, that play a role in the protective mechanisms of the body; *albumins*, that play an essential role in maintaining the exchange of fluid between the blood and the body tissues.

prothrombin. A substance present in the fluid part of the blood that is fundamental for the clotting of blood. Without this substance bleeding would never stop. Prothrombin is formed in the liver through the action of vitamin K. In the presence of calcium and thromboplastin, a substance produced when skin or other tissue is injured, prothrombin is converted to *thrombin*. Thrombin, in turn, converts *fibrinogen*, one of the plasma proteins, into *fibrin*. Fibrin is essentially a long, threadlike tissue that forms a network in which the red and white blood cells are caught to jell and form a clot.

protoplasm. The essential material of all living cells, thick and fluid-like, upon which all the vital functions of the cell depend.

Protozoa. A large family of microscopic, one-celled organisms, the simplest form of animal life. Many of these produce disease in man, including the *amoeba* that causes dysentery; the *plasmodium*, that causes malaria; the *leishmania*, that causes *kala-azar*; and the *trypanosoma*, that causes sleeping sickness.

prurigo (*proo-righ'goh*). A disease of the skin that comes on slowly, lasts a long time, and is characterized by small, pale bumps and severe itching. These bumps are very deep in the skin and are particularly prevalent in the limbs.

pruritus (*proo-righ'tuhss*). Itching, a symptom rather than a disease in itself. —*p. ani.* A long-standing, intense itching around the anus, most often occurring in men. May be due to hemorrhoids, local infection with fungi, allergy, and very often to psychological disorders. —*p. vulvae.* Itching of the vagina and the surrounding tissues that may result in thickening, shrinking of tissues, and at times even cancer. Due to many causes, and very frequently psychological in origin.

pseudocyesis (*soo-doh-sigh-ee'sihss*). Phantom pregnancy. All of the signs and symptoms including the protrusion of the abdomen may be present. Caused by a psychological disturbance.

pseudohermaphrodite (*soo-doh-huhr-maaf'roh-dight*). An individual with deformed external genitals that take on the appearance of the genitals of one sex, while the sex glands are those of the other sex. These are the cases who, by operation, are transformed from man to woman, or woman to man.

psittacosis (*siht-tuh-koh'sihss*). A disease of sudden onset with high fever, caused by a virus transmitted to man through parrots. Pneumonia is commonly part of the picture.

psoas (*soh'uhss*). The general name of two muscles, *p. major* and *p. minor*, that arise from the spine in the low back, swing around the side, and attach themselves to the thigh bone. Its function is to bend the hipjoint, drawing the trunk down and forward.

psoriasis (*saw-righ'uh-sihss*). A disease of slow inception, unknown cause, and long duration involving the skin, characterized by patches of red that are covered with silver white scales. Affects particularly the scalp, hairless surface of the forearms, hands, and calves. Psoriasis may involve any part of the body. It tends to recur particularly during times of emotional stress. Treatment is often unsatisfactory.

psychiatry. That branch of medicine that deals with diseases of the mind and their treatment.

psychoanalysis. A method for exploring the emotional patterns and their origins, and the thinking processes. Developed by Sigmund Freud. Psychoanalysis is used in the treatment of a wide variety of emotional disturbances, particularly those known as the *neuroses*. The basic means is *free association*, which is the patient's speaking whatever comes into his mind. In this fashion much information of which the patient himself is unaware is brought out. From this information, both the patient and the analyst learn the reasons for the direction in life the patient has taken.

psychodynamics. The various causes and their relationships involved in the mental and emotional activity of the individual.

psychology. The science that deals with the various functions of the mind, such as memory, intelligence, sensation, perception, and, in the larger sense, the behavior of an individual, man or animal, in relation to the world about him. *—abnormal p.* The study of irregular mental activity, such as illusions, delusions, hallucinations.

psychoneurosis. A general term for a large number of mental disorders, all of which, as far as is known, are not due to physical disease. These disorders are all characterized by various emotional states, the degree of which is disproportionate to reality and play a concealed but protective role in the emotional life of the patient. Anxieties, fears, obsessions, and multiple physical disabilities are common in psychoneurosis.

psychopath. A person with no grasp of moral responsibility, who is continually in conflict with accepted social behavior, and frequently the law.

psychosexual. Referring to the emotional and mental aspects of sex in contrast to the physical and glandular aspects. Example: impotence in a man for which there is no physical reason is a psychosexual disturbance.

psychosis. A disease of the mind in which the individual loses practically complete touch with reality. *—alcoholic p.* Due to alcoholism. *—arteriosclerotic p.* Due to hardening of the arteries, particularly in the brain. *—manic-depressive p.* Of unknown cause, characterized by states of markedly increased activity both mental and physical with an extraordinary sense of well-being and great self-regard; and other states of severe depression, immobility and melancholy. Also known as *affective-reaction p.*

psychosomatic. Relates to a conception in medicine that the mind and the body are not separate entities, but are rather different expressions of the same underlying unity.

psychosurgery. An operation on the brain performed in certain types of mental disorders in which the fore part of the brain is cut across, thus severing the pathways that serve to connect higher mental processes and the emotions. This operation is used with a great deal of success in certain cases that formerly were considered hopeless.

psychotherapy. Treatment of mental disorders by psychological means, among them suggestion. The latter technique, directed at removal of symptoms, is applied while patient is awake or under hypnosis. Suggestion is to be differentiated from *psychoanalysis,* which attempts to get at the cause of symptoms rather than merely relieve them.

ptomaine (*toh'mayn*). A compound that is the result of the breakdown by germs of decayed or dead animal matter.

ptosis (*toh'sihss*). The falling down or the depression of an organ, as a drooping upper lid, through the paralysis or shrinking of the muscle that lifts the lid.

ptyalin (*tigh'uh-lihn*). An enzyme in saliva that begins the process of breaking down carbohydrates, as starch, in the mouth.

ptyalorrhea (*tigh-uh-lawr-ree'uh*). An excessive flow of saliva.

ptysis (*tigh'sihss*). The act of spitting.

puberty. That period in the developing young person when the sex glands have matured to the point where reproduction can occur. Usually appears between the 11th and 14th years and is characterized by the appearance of hair in the region of the genital and in the armpits, and, in the male, by a deepening of the voice and emission of semen; in the female, by the appearance of the monthly period.

pubes (*pyou'beez*). The hairy region just above the genital.

puerperium (*pyou-uhr-pee'rih-um*). The state of a woman who has just been delivered of a child, or the period from the time of delivery to the time when the womb has returned to its normal size, approximately six to eight weeks.

pulse. Arteries have elastic walls that stretch with each expression of blood from the heart into the blood vessel system. When the heart is in the period of rest, immediately after expulsion of blood, the artery walls relax. This change from a stretched to a relaxed condition of the artery wall constitutes the pulse. Ordinarily the pulse is counted at the wrist, the *radial artery*. It may be taken over any artery that can be felt—at the neck, temple, inside the upper arm, toward the inside of the upper part of the thigh, and in other areas.

puncture. A hole made by insertion of a pointed instrument. —*lumbar p.* The puncture of the canal in the spine in the low back made in order to remove spinal fluid for certain diagnostic tests or for the introduction of medication. Also called *spinal p.*. —*sternal p.* Puncture of the breastbone with a large-bore, hollow needle in order to remove some of the bone marrow for examination to determine the presence of certain diseases.

purpura (*puhr'pyou-ruh*). A condition in which there is bleeding into the skin, the lining tissues of various organs and body cavities, and within organs themselves. This condition appears without cause or very slight injury. —*idiopathic thrombocytopenic p.* A disease in which first very tiny and then larger hemorrhages occur on the limbs and in successive crops over a great part of the skin surface. Bleeding may occur in lining tissues or from body cavities to the outside. Among other findings in this condition is a decrease in the number of platelets or thrombocytes in the blood. Also called *Werlhof's disease.* —*nonthrombopenic p.* Here bleeding from the intestines occurs, associated with nausea, vomiting, diarrhea, and pain in the abdomen. Also called *Henoch's disease.* —*rheumatic p.* A type that is accompanied by severe arthritis. Also called *Schoenlein's disease.* —*symptomatic p.* A type that comes on with either infectious diseases or cancerous tumors, kidney disease, and other blood diseases. May be the result of drug allergy. Also called *secondary p.*

purulent (*pyour'uh-luhnt*). Made of, containing, or manufacturing pus.

pus. A yellow or greenish, creamlike liquid produced in an area of inflammation and composed mostly of white blood cells and serum. The color of pus varies with the germ that stimulates its production.

pustule. A small, raised area of the skin containing pus, as a pimple from which pus can be expressed.

putrefaction. Rotting; decaying. The disintegration of matter brought about by certain germs, accompanied by the production of gasses, acids, and other poisonous substances, all of which have a disagreeable odor.

pyelitis (*pigh-uh-ligh'tihss*). Inflammation of the pelvis of the kidney. The pelvis is a large, basin-shaped part of the middle of the exterior of the kidney, actually the expanded upper portion of the passageway (ureter) for urine from the kidney to the bladder.

pyelogram. An X-ray of the pelvis of the kidney and the ureter that have been filled with a solution not permitting the passage of X-rays. This opacity serves to outline the pelvis and ureter on the film.

pyelonephritis (*pigh-uh-loh-nih-frigh'tihss*). Inflammation of the kidney and its pelvis, usually due to an infection that comes up the ureter.

pygmalionism (*pihg-may'lee-uh-nihsm*). An emotionally distorted state in which an individual falls in love with a creation of his own.

pyloroplasty (*pigh-law'roh-plaass-tih*). The exit from the stomach is a narrow passageway that contains muscle in its wall, the *pylorus*. Often an ulcer forms in this region, causing the muscle to squeeze down and narrow, or to close off the passageway. The operation necessary to reestablish the passageway is called pyloroplasty.

pylorus (*pigh-law'ruhss*). Specifically applied to the muscle and lining tissue that surround the opening between the stomach and the first part of the small intestine; also refers to the lower portion of the stomach.

pyoderma. Any inflammation of the skin that produces pus, as large numbers of boils or carbuncles.

pyrethrum flowers. The flowers of a plant of the chrysanthemum family, a cousin of ragweed, used in powdered form as an insecticide and in an ointment for the treatment of scabies. Not uncommonly the cause of allergic symptoms.

pyrexia. Fever.

pyrogen (*pigh'roh-jehn*). Not infrequently when injections or drips are given into a vein, the patient develops fever. This fever is caused by certain bacteria present in water that are killed during the process of distilling the water. The dead bodies of these bacteria are believed to cause the fever and are called pyrogens.

pyruvic acid. An acid that is normally produced in the body during a stage in the breaking down of carbohydrates or proteins. When there is a deficiency in one of the vitamin-B complex (*thiamine*), pyruvic acid may appear in excess quantity in the blood and tissues.

pyuria. Pus in the urine.

Q

quadriceps (*kwahd'ruh-sehps*). A four-headed muscle situated on the front part of the thigh, that acts to elevate the thigh.

quadripara (*kwahd-rihp'uh-ruh*). A woman bearing or who has borne a fourth child.

quadriplegia. Paralysis of both arms and legs.

quarantine. 1. The restriction of people who have been exposed to a communicable disease for a period of time equivalent to the incubation period of the disease to which they have been exposed. 2. The detention place of such people. 3. The detention of ships or passengers from places suspected of certain disease for the purpose of disinfection.

quinsy. An inflammation of the tonsil and the tissue surrounding the tonsil, usually leading to an abscess. Also called *peritonsillar abscess.*

quintipara (*kwihn-tihp'uh-ruh*). A woman who is bearing or who has borne a fifth child.

R

rabid. Relating to rabies or infected with rabies.

rabies (*ray'beez*). An infectious disease of sudden onset due to a virus transmitted to other animals and man by the bite of an infected animal. Any animal may carry the disease, but it occurs most frequently in the cat, wolf, and dog. The virus causing this disease is particularly attracted to the nervous system, and is found in the saliva of the infected individual. In man there are ordinarily three stages of rabies: the *first* in which there is obvious ill-health, restlessness, and fear; the *second* in which the individual becomes extremely overactive and has spasms of the muscles that control swallowing and breathing; and the *third* that begins with drooling of saliva and ends fatally with a paralysis eventually striking the muscles controlling breathing. —*r. prophylaxis.* The daily injection of the person exposed to rabies with vaccine made from ground-up spinal cords of rabbits infected with the virus. This treatment continues for 14 days, the first injection of material from a cord that has been dried for 14 days, and each succeeding injection of a cord one day fresher than the preceding.

rachitic (*ruh-kiht'ihk*). Resembling, produced by, or affected with, rickets.

radial. 1. Proceeding in a divergent direction from a common center, as the spokes of a wheel from its hub. 2. Relating to the radius, the bone on the thumb side of the forearm.

radiation. 1. The act of diverging from a central point as the radiation of light, or having the appearance of rays. 2. The use of X-rays or radium in treatment.

radicular. Relating to a root, particularly to the root of a spinal nerve that is in close proximity to the spinal column.

radiculitis (*raa-dihk-yuh-ligh'tihss*). Inflammation of a nerve root.

radiograph. An X-ray film. Also called *roentgenogram.*

radiography. The making of X-ray pictures.

radiologist. A doctor who specializes in the use of X-ray and/or radium in determining the cause and treatment of disease.

radiology. That branch of medicine that deals with the making of diagnoses and treatment of disease by X-ray and radium.

radiopaque (*ray-dih-oh-payk'*). Not permitting the passage of X-rays.

radiosensitivity. The quality by which tissues or organisms are affected by X-ray exposure.

radiotherapeutic. Relating to the use of X-ray or radium for treatment.

ragweed. A weed whose pollen is responsible for a great proportion of fall hay fever in the U. S. in the area east of the Rocky Mountains. Ragweed produces pollen from the middle of August to October.

râle (*raal*). An abnormal sound usually heard through the stethoscope over the lungs or bronchi. Classified as coarse and fine, sometimes as moist or dry. A râle indicates that something is not right within the air passages. *—crepitant r.* A fine, crackling sound that resembles the rubbing together of hairs. This sound is not invariably an indication of disease, but may be heard when unaccustomed deep breaths are taken. *—rhoncus r.* A very coarse sound that usually comes from the large air-tubes and may be heard all over the chest. *—sibilant r.* A hissing or whistling sound of high pitch usually heard when the very small breathing tubes are in spasm. *—sonorous r.* A snoring sound heard in cases of spasm of the small breathing tubes.

ramus (*ray'muhss*). 1. A branch of an artery, vein, or nerve. 2. A projecting, branchlike part, usually slender, from a large bone, as the ramus of the lower jaw; a slender, lathlike extension of bone from the angle of the jaw to the joint of the jaw directly in front of the ear.

rate. The speed or frequency of a process measured against a standard. *—sedimentation r.* ESR is the abbreviation for *erythrocyte sedimentation rate*, the rate at which red blood cells settle out of a specimen of blood to which sodium citrate has been added to prevent clotting. In certain diseases, such as infections in general and rheumatic fever, this rate is markedly increased.

ratio. The relative size of two quantities. For instance, the odds quoted in racing are a ratio, two to one, three to one, one to five. —*albumin-globulin r.* Normally in the serum of the blood, the proteins, albumin, and globulin, are in the ratio of 1.3-1.8 to 1. Changes in this proportion indicate certain general types of disease and disturbance.

rationalization. Making an idea, judgment, action appear reasonable when it is evidently irrational. This process arises in the unconscious and is aimed at making unconscious urges appear reasonable.

ray. A beam of light or a stream of tiny particles. —*Roentgen rays.* X-rays. —*ultraviolet r.* Invisible light rays that tan the skin and destroy many types of bacteria.

Raynaud's disease. A disease, the result of disturbance of the nervous system, causing spasm of the very small blood vessels. Raynaud's disease begins suddenly and affects the fingers, toes, and at times the lips, nose, chin, and ears. There are three stages: severe pain, numbness, coldness, and paleness of the affected parts; parts become blue or black, the pain is intense, blisters may appear; parts may drop off.

recidivation (*rih-sihd-ih-vay'shuhn*). 1. The recurrence of a disease. 2. Relapsing into crime.

recrudescence. An increase in the symptoms of a disease after it has disappeared or been markedly reduced.

rectocele (*rehk'toh-seel*). The bulging of the rectum into the vagina, frequently occurring in women who have had one or more children.

rectofistula. A longitudinal, painful crack in the lining membrane of the rectum.

rectoscope. An instrument that is inserted into the rectum in order to visualize it.

rectum. The lower part of the large intestine that ends in the anus.

reflex. A specific type of response to a stimulus that is entirely involuntary. —*abdominal r.* Drawing the fingernail across the skin of the abdomen causes a contraction of the muscles. This reflex can be seen by movement of the navel in the direction of the finger.   *—Achilles tendon r.* When the tendon at the back of the ankle is struck a sharp blow, the foot will bend, toes pointing down, due to the calf muscles going into spasm.   *—ankle clonus r.* If pressure is made against the sole of the foot, the calf muscles will contract and relax rapidly, causing the foot to move up and down in rapid succession.   *—Babinski r.* In certain diseases or injuries of the nervous system, stroking the sole of the foot will result in the large toe bending up.   *—patellar r.* Striking the tendon just below the kneecap when the leg is crossed upon the other will result in a quick jerking forward of the lower leg. Also called the *knee jerk.*

refraction. The process of determining errors in vision by placing lenses of various strength in a frame in front of the eye to visualize an eye chart with lines of letters of various size twenty feet away.

refractory. Resistant to treatment; resistant to stimulation.

regeneration. The growth or repair of structures or tissues lost through disease or injury. Examples: the growth of skin over a small wound, the re-growth of a nail that has fallen out.

region. A natural or arbitrary division of the body.   *—abdominal r.* An arbitrary region marked out by two horizontal lines, the upper passing across the front of the trunk at the level of the flare of the ribs, the lower at the level of the top of the hipbone. The vertical lines on each side extend from the middle of the thigh into the ribs.   *—anterior cubital r.* The fold of the elbows.   *—popliteal r.* The region of the fold of the knee.   *—scapular r.* The region over the shoulder blades.   *—sternal r.* The region of the breastbone.

regression. It is believed that the individual in his development to maturity as a social being passes through a number of stages each specifically related to the conscious and unconscious handling of the sexual urges. When at any stage there is a turning back to an earlier stage, regression is said to have taken place.

regurgitation. 1. A backflow of blood into the heart through a valve that is defective. 2. The effortless return of food from the stomach, in this way unlike vomiting.

reinfection. A return of infection with the same kind of germ.

relapse. The return of symptoms after a disease seems to have been cured.

relapsing fever. The general name for a group of infectious diseases caused by certain spiral-shaped germs transmitted to man by lice or ticks. Characterized by a sudden onset with chills, fever, enlargement of the spleen, pain in the back and legs, delirium, and at times convulsions. Symptoms disappear rapidly and recur after a week or more. May repeat two to six times. Also called *tick fever, louse fever, famine fever*.

relax. To make limber or less tense.

remission. The disappearance of symptoms of a disease, or the time that it takes for this action to occur.

rennin (*rehn'ihn*). A constituent of the digestive juice, manufactured by the stomach, that curdles milk. This curdling represents the first step in the breakdown of the protein in milk.

repression. The pushing down into unconsciousness of unacceptable feelings, emotions, ideas. This pushed-down material continues active in the unconscious and requires constant expenditure of energy to keep it there. The repressed material often emerges from the unconscious in the form of symptoms. Example: a son's hatred for his father is repressed but emerges as a hatred for some superior in no way related to the father.

resect. To remove surgically a piece of tissue or organ, as in stomach resection.

resistance. The constant attempt at preventing unwanted or painful material from emerging into consciousness. This activates repression. *See also* REPRESSION.

resolution. The subsiding of inflammation, as the resolution of a boil when it disappears with or without the discharge of pus.

respiration. 1. The exchange of gases between an organism and the medium in which it lives, as the exchange of carbon dioxide for oxygen by a single-celled plant or animal (a germ). 2. The act of taking air into and expelling it from the lungs. This act consists of *inspiration*, the taking of air into the lungs; and *expiration*, the expelling of the remnant air and various gases given up by the body, as carbon dioxide. The air exhaled contains less oxygen and more carbon dioxide than the air inhaled. The normal amount of air taken into and given out of the lungs during the average respiration is about a pint. The amount that can be inhaled in addition by a deep inhalation is a quart and a half. The air remaining in the lungs after a forceful exhalation is about a quart and a half. The amount of air that can be forcibly exhaled after a deep and forcible inhalation is called the *vital capacity* and is about three and a half quarts.

restitution. The act of restoring.

resuscitation. The prevention of death by asphyxia through artificial respiration, as in the case of a person unconscious due to near-drowning.

retention. The act of holding back, as the holding of urine in the bladder due to some obstruction to urination.

reticulocyte (*rih-tihk'yuh-loh-sight*). A young, undeveloped red blood cell with a fine interior network. Normally present in the blood stream in small numbers. When present in greater numbers it indicates an overactivity of the red blood-cell forming organs, seen as a response to liver treatment in pernicious anemia.

retina (*reht'ih-nuh*). The innermost of the three coats of the eyeball, actually an expansion of the head of the nerve of sight that enters the eyeball from behind. The retina receives light sensation and transforms it into nervous impulses that are then sent along the nerve of sight to the brain for translation into vision.

retinitis. Inflammation of the retina caused by a number of conditions, as diabetes, leukemia, pregnancy, kidney disease, and syphilis. Results in a definite interference with vision.

retinoscopy (*reht-ih-nahss'kuh-pih*). A method of determining the degree of far or nearsightedness of the eye. The instrument used is the retinoscope, a mirror on a handle. Light is directed from the mirror into the patient's pupil. The mirror is rotated. If the shadow in the illuminated pupil moves in the same direction as the mirror, the eye is farsighted. Proper lenses are placed before the eye until movement of the shadow is abolished, constituting the correction of the eye. If the shadow in the illuminated pupil moves in the opposite direction to the mirror, the eye is nearsighted and proper lenses are placed in front of the eye until the shadow remains stationary.

retraction. The act of drawing back, as a tendon that when cut pulls back, resembling the snapping back of a stretched rubber band when one end is released.

retractor. A surgical instrument used to hold back the edges of a wound so that the surgeon may have access to deeper parts. Ordinarily made of a handle with a small right-angle extension.

retropharynx. The back wall of the throat. Easily seen in a mirror when the mouth is opened wide.

retroversion. A turning back on itself, as tipping back of the womb toward the spine.

rhabdomyoma (*raab-doh-migh-oh'muh*). A tumor, usually not dangerous to life, composed of tissue from which develops striped muscle (muscle under control of the will and heart muscle).

rhagades (*raag'uh-deez*). Cracks in skin that has lost its ability to stretch through infection, inflammation, or tumor growth. Seen in syphilis and other conditions.

rheumatism. Generally indicates diseases of nerves, bones, joints, muscles, and tendons accompanied by discomfort and physical incapacity. —*acute rheumatic fever*. A disease of sudden onset with high fever, swelling and pain migrating from joint to joint. Damage of the heart and particularly its valves is very common. The joints are never permanently injured. Although the cause is not definitely known, it is related to streptococcus infections, particularly of the throat, and is primarily a disease of childhood, attacking girls more often than boys. —*gonorrheal r.* Arthritis due to infection with the germ that produces gonorrhea, *Neisseria gonorrheae.* —*pallindromic r.* A condition characterized by attacks of severe arthritis with swelling, redness, and pain, usually of one joint at a time. The attack lasts for a few hours or days after which the symptoms completely disappear. Cause is not known; may be an allergy.

RH factor. An element in the blood so called because it was first found in the blood cells of the Rhesus monkey. *RH positive* and *RH negative* are terms that indicate the presence or absence of this element in the blood. When the father is RH positive and the mother RH negative, the RH positive factor is transmitted to the developing infant within the mother's womb. This factor stimulates in the mother production of certain protective substances (known as antibodies) against the RH factor. These antibodies pass from the mother's blood through the afterbirth into the blood of the developing infant and destroy its red blood cells, an action that may result in abortion. If the child is born it may die of jaundice and anemia. It is necessary to know the RH character of blood before giving a transfusion since RH positive blood given to an RH negative subject may result in serious injury.

rhinitis. Inflammation of the lining tissue of the interior of the nose. —*acute r.* The common cold. —*allergic r.* Often called hay fever; may be caused by allergy to material other than pollen. —*atrophic r.* Inflammation followed by permanent shrinking of the mucous membrane within the nose. —*syphilitic r.* May come on late in syphilis accompanied by sores in the nose, decay of the nose bones, and foul discharge. —*tuberculous r.* Associated with tuberculosis elsewhere in the body, usually the lungs, manifested by ulcerating sores in the nose and decay of the nose bone. —*vasomotor r.* Another name for year-around hay fever. Also called *allergic r., perennial allergic r., perennial allergic coryza.*

rhinologist. A specialist in diseases of the nose.

rhinology. That branch of medicine dealing with the structure, functions, diseases and their treatment, of the nose.

rhinophyma (*righ-noh-figh'muh*). A lasting inflammation of the skin of the nose giving it the appearance of a reddish enlarged lump, usually disfiguring and often following prolonged, excessive use of alcohol. Also called *whiskey nose* and *toper's nose.*

rhinorrhaphy (*righ-nawr'ruh-fih*). A plastic operation on the nose to reduce its size and to reconstruct it.

rhinoscleroma. A tumor growth of stony hardness involving the nostrils and surrounding parts.

rhomboideus (*rahm-boy'dih-uhss*). The name of a group of muscles that arise from the spinal column of the lower half of the neck and the upper half of the chest and attach to the inner edge of the shoulder blade.

rhonchus (*rahn'kuhss*). A rough, low-pitched snoring type of abnormal sound heard in the chest, caused by the accumulation of mucus in the large breathing tubes or windpipe. Not uncommonly heard in certain stages of asthma.

rib. One of the twelve pairs of curved, flat bones forming the chest wall. —*cervical ribs.* On occasion a riblike extension of bone is found arising from one of the vertebrae in the neck, a *cervical rib*, that may cause trouble by pressing on a large network of nerves. Such pressure may result in pain and/or paralysis of the arm on the affected side. It is often necessary surgically to remove such a rib. —*false r.* The upper seven pairs of ribs are attached to the breast bone in front by gristle, *the true ribs.* The lower five pairs of ribs are not, and are called *the false ribs.* The eighth, ninth, and tenth pair are attached to a common piece of gristle that then attaches itself to the breast bone. The eleventh and twelfth pair of ribs are not attached to either gristle or the breast bone but their front ends are free, and these are *the floating ribs.*

Rickettsia. The name of a group of germs smaller than bacteria but larger than viruses, usually carried by spiders, ticks, fleas, and lice, and which produces a number of diseases in man, as typhus, trench fever, Rocky Mountain spotted fever, tsutsugamushi disease, rickettsialpox, and others.

rickettsialpox. A disease caused by one of the rickettsial germs characterized by headache, fever, chills, enlargement of the glands, and a small pimple at the site of the bite followed by a rash all over the body. Usually a self-limited disease without any complications or fatalities, transmitted by a mite carried by a mouse.

rigidity. Stiffness, immobility. A state of constant spasm of the muscle. —*cogwheel r.* The rigidity of muscles seen in *paralysis agitans* where the limb remains stiff in the position placed, much like a cogwheel.

rigor. Derived from the Latin meaning stiffness. —*r. mortis.* The stiffening of muscles that takes place after death.

ringworm. *See* DERMATOPHYTOSIS.

risus (*righ'suhss*). A laugh or a grin. —*r. sardonicus.* Peculiar distortion of the face into a sardonic grin, produced by spasm of the muscles about the mouth, occurring in tetanus and strychnine poisoning. Also called *r. caninus* (the dog's grin).

Rocky Mountain spotted fever. A disease occurring throughout the Western Hemisphere characterized by fever and rash caused by a germ, *Rickettsia rickettsi*, transmitted to man by several types of ticks.

roentgenogram (*rehnt'guhn-uh-graam*). An X-ray picture.

roentgenologist (*rehnt-guh-nahl'uh-jihst*). A physician who specializes in the use of X-rays for diagnosis and treatment. Also called *radiologist.*

roentgenotherapy. Treatment with X-rays.

rose fever. Hay fever, due to the pollen of grasses, that in the United States starts in May and ends in July.

roseola. A rose-colored eruption, as *r. cholerica*, an eruption that at times appears in cholera. —*r. typhosa*, an eruption seen in typhus or typhoid fever.

rubefacient (*roo-bih-fay'shuhnt*). Any agent that produces redness of the skin, the result of bringing blood into the surface blood vessels, as when a mustard plaster is applied.

rubella. *German measles.* A mild, contagious disease of short duration that sets in with sore throat, slight fever, and a reddish eruption that usually disappears in a day or two. Also called *French measles, epidemic roseola.*

rubeola. Measles.

rubor (*roo'bawr*). Redness due to inflammation seen around most infected or inflamed areas.

runaround. An infection that extends all the way around a finger or toenail.

rupture. 1. The tearing of a part by force, as a ruptured stomach, a ruptured spleen. 2. A hernia.

S

sac. A pouch. A baglike covering. —*conjunctival s.* The pouch formed in the very lowest aspect of the under-surface of the eyelid where the lining tissue extends from the lid onto the eyeball. —*hernial s.* The protrusion of the lining tissue of the abdominal cavity that contains the part or organ that is pushing out. This sac is formed by the gradual pressure of the intestine against a defect in the abdominal wall present from birth. —*pericardial s.* The pouch around the heart formed by its outer layer, the *pericardium.*

sacculation (*saak-yuh-lay'shuhn*). 1. The state of being divided into small sacs. 2. The formation of small sacs.

sacroiliac. Relating to the juncture of the hipbone and the lower part of the spine. Used loosely to indicate an inflammation of this joint that may produce sciatica and pain over the low back extending into the thigh.

sacrum. A flattened bone that is a union of five vertebrae situated just below the small of the back and uniting the two hipbones behind.

sadism. A sexual perversion in which pleasure is derived from inflicting pain on another.

St. Anthony's fire. An obsolete name for *erysipelas, gangrene,* or poisoning with ergot. A common characteristic of this condition is a bright-red appearance of the skin.

St. Vitus' dance. A condition in which purposeless motions are performed by various muscles of the body at times giving the patient the appearance of dancing. Also called *chorea.*

saline (*say'lighn*). 1. Saltlike. 2. Containing salt; commonly refers to a salt solution given by vein.

saliva. The secretions of the various glands in the mouth, particularly the salivary glands. Saliva is a thin, tasteless fluid that moistens and lubricates food, thus facilitates swallowing, and helps in talking. Saliva contains an important enzyme, *ptyalin,* that starts off the process of breaking down starches into less complicated substances.

salivation. An excess secretion of saliva produced by certain nervous conditions and mercury or pilocarpine poisoning. In mercury poisoning, loosening of the teeth and ulcers in the mouth may appear in addition to salivation.

Salmonella (*saal-muh-nehl'luh*). A type of germ, also known as *paratyphoid bacilli,* that causes acute stomach upsets as *food poisoning.* There are about 13 known kinds.

salpingectomy. The surgical removal of a tube of the womb.

salpingitis (*saal-pihn-jigh'tihss*). 1. Inflammation of the tubes between ovary and womb. 2. Inflammation of the tube that runs from the middle ear to the throat just behind the tonsil.

salpingo-oophoritis (*saal-pihn-goh-oh-oh-faw-righ'tihss*). Inflammation of the tube of the womb and the ovary.

saltpeter. Potassium nitrate. Popularly believed to reduce sexual desire and the power of erection of the penis.

sanatorium. A place for the treatment of diseases of long duration. Particularly a private hospital or a place having natural elements, as mineral baths, to relieve symptoms.

sand fly. The common name for the tribe of flying insects known as *Phlebotomus*. Transmits a variety of diseases to man.

sanguine. 1. Bloody or resembling blood. 2. Active, hopeful.

saphenous vein (*suh-fee'nuhss*). Either of two veins of the leg immediately under the skin, the *great* or *long saphenous vein* and the *small* or *short saphenous vein*, commonly involved in *varicose veins*.

sapphism (*saaf'izm*). Lesbianism; homosexuality in the female.

sarcoidosis. A disease of unknown cause affecting mostly young adults, involving lymph glands, lungs, skin, the far ends of bones particularly of the hands and feet, the eye, and other parts of the body. Lasts a long time with flare-ups of fever and general sickness. Although recovery may take place, death eventually results. Called by many other names, such as *Beck's sarcoid, Besnier's-Beck disease.*

sarcoma. A cancerous tumor of serious nature. There are many varieties of sarcoma named according to the specific tissue from which they arise or from the type of changes induced.

saturnism. Lead poisoning of gradual onset and long duration. Also called *plumbism.*

satyriasis (*saat-ih-righ'uh-sihss*). Excessive sexual desire in the male.

saucerize. In certain infections of bone, as *osteomyelitis*, where pieces of bone are eaten away, the cavity resulting has many sharp angles and overhanging walls that prevent the soft tissues from healing. To saucerize is to shape the bone cavity smoothly and thus to permit healing.

scabicide (*skay'bih-sighd*). Any agent that kills the insect producing scabies.

scabies (*skay'beez*). A contagious infestation of the skin by an insect, *Sarcoptes scabiei*. The female insect burrows beneath the skin to lay its eggs, causing irritation and intense itching (especially at night). Although the infestation may spread all over the body, it is most common in the webs of the fingers and, girdlelike, around the abdomen. Before scratching has camouflaged the appearance of the inflammation, small black dots in regular or irregular pattern may be seen in these areas. These dots are the burrows of the insect.

scalenus (*skuh-lee'nuhss*). The general name of three muscles that arise in the vertebrae of the neck and attach to the first two ribs. Their function is to bend the neck from one side to the other, and to help in breathing under circumstances when breathing is difficult.

scalpel. A knife used in surgery with a long, firm handle, and a short, rounded, or straight blade that may be pointed or blunt at the end.

scaphoid. 1. Boat-shaped. 2. A boat-shaped bone of the ankle and the wrist. Also called *navicular*.

scapula (*skaap'yuh-luh*). The shoulder blade. A flat, large, triangular-shaped bone at the back of the shoulders.

scarlatina. Another name for scarlet fever.

scarlet fever. A contagious disease, especially of childhood, coming on suddenly with fever, vomiting, chills, sore throat, inflammation of the glands in the neck, and (within one to five days) a pin-point or scarlet eruption. In the beginning, the tongue is heavily coated, and bright red at the tip and edges. Shortly thereafter the coating disappears and the tongue becomes red and swollen with prominent elevations giving it the appearance of a strawberry. When the eruption appears, all the symptoms become worse. After five to six days all fade and the eruption begins to scale off. The kidneys are very commonly involved as a complication. Scarlet fever is caused by a streptococcus and is transmitted from man to man in the same manner as a common cold. Once the organism arrives in the susceptible person, the symptoms come on within several hours to a week.

scatology (*skuh-tahl'uh-jih*). The study of body excretions, as urine and feces.

schistosomiasis (*shihss-tuh-soh-migh'uh-sihss*). 1. Infestation with a type of blood fluke called *Schistosoma*. 2. An inflammation of the skin characterized by small elevations with or without pus, occurring in people wading or swimming in fresh water lakes of northern U. S. and Canada. Schistosomiasis is due to the penetration of the skin by the young forms of a blood fluke. These blood flukes are parasites of snails. The condition in this hemisphere is generally mild and disappears of itself. In Africa, Japan, China, South America, and the West Indies the disease takes on a much more serious form, involving the urinary bladder, stomach, intestines, and liver, and is frequently fatal. Also called *swimmer's itch*, *bilharziasis*.

schizophrenia (*skihz-uh-free'nih-uh*). A form of insanity characterized by a lack of feeling, unpredictable behavior, moods that are not appropriate to reality, and a gradual mental deterioration. It often ends in complete withdrawal from the world of reality into fantasies that the individual erects.

sciatica. A disease characterized by pain, numbness, tingling, tenderness to the touch along the course of the sciatic nerve that runs from low on the buttock down the back of the thigh into the heel. Sciatica is due to inflammation or injury of the nerve and may result in shrinkage and wasting of the muscles of the thigh and leg.

scirrhus (*skihr'uhss*). A cancer that is extremely hard to the touch.

sclera (*sklih'ruh*). The outermost coat of the eyeball composed of tough tissues. In front it becomes the white and the transparent part of the eye.

sclerectomy. The surgical removal of a part of the sclera.

scleritis. Inflammation of the outer coat of the eye.

scleroderma. A disease of the skin, of unknown cause, in which patches or large areas become extremely hardened and take on a mottled color. At times the muscles beneath the skin show the same changes.

sclerosis. A general name for the hardening of a part by overgrowth of tough, fibrous tissue. Applied especially to the nervous system where hardening may occur through deterioration of the nerve elements and their replacement by tough, fibrous tissue; and to arteries whose coats become thickened and hard and accumulate calcium and fats. —*multiple s.* A condition of unknown cause in which patches of hardening occur in different parts of the nervous system. The chief symptoms are monotonous speech occurring in syllables, rapid movements of the eyes, weakness of the muscles, and trembling of the legs and arms when motion is attempted. —*posterolateral s.* Affects chiefly a specialized area of the spinal cord, characterized by numbness and tingling, loss of the vibratory sense, loss of co-ordination of muscles, and spasms of muscles. Occurs very frequently in the course of pernicious anemia.

sclerotomy. The surgical incision of the outer coat of the eyeball. —*anterior s.* An incision made through the top and front part of the white of the eye into the front chamber of the eye in order to reduce the pressure within the eyeball in cases of glaucoma.

scoliosis. Curvature of the spine to one side or the other caused by a defect in the development of the spine from birth, faulty posture, and various diseases that affect the spine or the muscles attached to the spine.

scotoma. A blind spot on the retina; an area on the retina that does not transmit light impulses to the brain.

scrofula (*skrahf'yuh-luh*). Tuberculosis of the lymph glands in the neck.

scrotum. The sac containing the testes composed of skin, muscle, an inner coat of tough tissue, and a lining tissue that is continuous with the outer lining of the testes.

scurvy. A disease produced by a lack of vitamin C, characterized by bleeding under the skin, from the lining tissues, and under the tough coat of tissue covering bone; by spongy gums; and by general weakness.

sebaceous (*sih-bay'shuhss*). Relating to, or excreting, sebum, the oily product of the oil glands of the skin.

seborrhea (*sehb-uh-ree'uh*). A disease of the oil glands of the skin characterized by an unusual amount of oil secretion or a change in the character of the oil secreted. This oil collects on the skin in the form of scales, crusts, or an oily coating.

sebum. The oily secretion of the oil glands of the skin.

secreta (*sih-kree'tuh*). The material produced and expelled by a gland or organ.

secrete. To form out of materials furnished by the blood, or to separate from the blood a certain substance known as a secretion.

secretion. 1. The act of forming from materials furnished by the blood a specific substance that is either eliminated from the body (excretion) or used in special procedures in the body. 2. The substance secreted. Examples: gastric secretion, the gastric juices; internal secretion, the product of the endocrine glands not thrown out onto a surface of the body, but absorbed into the blood (hormone).

section. 1. *n.* A dividing or cutting. 2. *n.* A cut or slice. 3. *v.* Cut through or divide. —*abdominal s.* A cutting into the abdominal cavity.

sedation. The production of a state of lesser activity and sensation.

sediment. The material that settles to the bottom of a fluid.

sella. A saddle. —*s. turcica.* The saddle of bone in the skull just behind the eyes in which the pituitary gland sits. Also called *Turkish saddle.*

semen. The fluid produced by the male organs of reproduction that carries the sperm.

semilunar. One of the bones of the wrist shaped like a half-moon.

semination. The introduction of semen into the vagina or womb.

senescence. Aging; growing old.

sepsis. A reaction of the body, usually with fever, the result of the action of infection with germs either by the germs themselves or by the product of the germs, such as toxins or both. —*puerperal s.* A complication of pregnancy due to infection in the womb by streptococci.

septicemia. A disease spread throughout the entire body produced by germs and their poisons in the blood. Also called blood poisoning.

septigravida (*sehp-tih-graav'ih-duh*). A woman pregnant for the seventh time.

septipara (*sehp-tihp'uh-ruh*). A woman who has borne seven children.

septum. A dividing wall between two spaces or cavities or parts; a partition. —*lingual s.* The partition running the length of the tongue that divides the tongue muscle into two halves. —*nasal s.* The partition that divides the nose into two chambers composed of bone above and gristle below. —*rectovaginal s.* The tissue partition that separates the rectum from the vagina.

sequela (*sih-kwee'luh*). An unusual condition occurring after a disease and directly or indirectly caused by it, as kidney disease following on scarlet fever.

sequestrum (*see-kwess'trum*). A dead piece of bone, partially or entirely detached, within a cavity, or wound, or abscess.

serology. That branch of science concerned with serum.

serosa. A specialized type of tissue that lines cavities of the body, such as the abdominal cavity, the chest cavity.

serpiginous (*suhr-pihj'ih-nuhss*). Having a snakelike shape, arched, creeping. Used in reference to skin eruptions.

serum. The straw-colored liquid that leaks out from a clot of blood or from a scabbed-over wound. Serum, obtained from the blood after clotting, is used for treatment. Within the serum are present many types of protective substances, if obtained from man or immunized animals. Thus there are *anti-dysentery serums, anti-plague serums, anti-RH serums,* and *normal human serum* used primarily for the treatment of general infection, burns, and shock.

sesamoid. A very small bone situated within a tendon that is subjected to much pressure, as the kneecap.

sex link. An hereditary characteristic that is attached to or transmitted through one or the other sex.

sextagravida (*sehks'tuh-graav-ih-duh*). A woman who is pregnant for the sixth time.

sextipara (*sehks-tihp'uh-ruh*). A woman who has borne six children.

shank. The leg from the knee to the ankle.

Shigella (*shih-ghehl'luh*). A class of germ belonging to the *Salmonella* tribe, producing dysentery.

shin. The sharp front margin of the leg. —*saber s.* A condition seen in the type of syphilis present from birth in which the shin is shaped like a saber, the bow forward.

shingles. *See* HERPES.

shock. 1. A medley of symptoms due essentially to injury, the result of an interference with circulation of blood and a fall in its pressure. May lead finally to the failure of circulation and death. Shock is classified according to its cause as surgical, burn, bleeding, injury; and according to the speed of its development, as *precipitous* or *delayed.* Also called *peripheral circulatory failure.* 2. Effect of drugs or electric shocks in shock therapy (*see* THERAPY). 3. A sudden and violent shaking of the emotional mechanism by some unexpected sensation or experience of paralyzing or revolting character.

shoulder. The region where the arm and the trunk join, formed by the union of the collarbone, the shoulderbone, the muscles, ligaments, and other soft tissue surrounding these bones.

sialagogue (*sigh-aal'uh-gahg*). 1. Causing a flow of saliva. 2. A drug that produces a flow of saliva.

sialorrhea (*sigh-uh-lawr-ree'uh*). The flowing of saliva.

sib. One of the progeny of the same parents; a brother or sister. Also called *sibling*.

siderosis (*sihd-uh-roh'sihss*). A gradually occurring inflammation of the lung due to the inhalation of dust containing iron or its salts. Appears in arc-welders and iron miners.

sight. 1. The act of seeing. 2. The particular sense concerned in seeing. —*aging s*. Presbyopia. —*day s*. Hemeralopia. —*far s*. Hypermetropia. —*short s*. Myopia. —*weak s*. Asthenopia.

sigmoid. 1. (*adj*.) Shaped like the letter S. 2. (*n*.) The lower part of the large bowel, shaped like the letter S, leading into the rectum.

sigmoidectomy. The surgical removal of a part or all of the S-shaped, lower portion of the large bowel.

sigmoidoscope. A long, tubular instrument arranged with a source of light that is inserted into the anus in order to inspect the lower portion of the large bowel.

sign. Objective evidence. Used particularly to differentiate the manifestations of disease that can be detected by the examiner from the symptoms felt by the patient. Example: headache is a symptom; limping is a sign.

silicosis (*sihl-ih-koh'sihss*). A generalized loss of the elastic quality of the lung accompanied by inflammation caused by prolonged inhalation of dust having a silica content. Occurs in quarry workers, stonecutters, stone-grinders.

sinapism (*sihn-uh-pihsm*). A mustard plaster.

sinew. A tendon.

sinister. Left; opposite of right.

sinus. 1. A cavity within a bone. 2. A cavity, recess, or pocket. 3. A large space containing blood, especially vein blood. 4. A channel that is producing pus. —*coronary s*. A sinus that drains blood from the veins within the heart-wall into the right atrium. —*paranasal s*. Air cavities that communicate with the nose and are lined by mucous membrane: the *frontal*, in the forehead just above the nose; the *ethmoid*, alongside the walls of the nose; the *sphenoid*, high up between the eyes under the pituitary gland; the *maxillary*, on either side of the nose under the eyes in the face.

sinusitis. Inflammation of any one or combination of paranasal sinuses.

situs (*sigh'tuhss*). A position. —*s. inversus.* A malformation in which the abdominal organs are located on the side of the body opposite to normal, as the liver on the left side, the spleen on the right.

skin. The body covering that consists of the *epidermis, scarf skin* or *cuticle;* and the *corium, true skin* or *derma.* The epidermis is the true protective layer composed of the tough tissue readily seen as skin. The corium consists of fibrous and elastic tissue and small patches of muscle that serve to erect the hairs. Underneath the skin is the fat, blood vessels, and sweat glands. The skin has appendages, as the nails; sweat, oil, milk glands; hair; and specialized nerve endings that transmit sensations of temperature, pain, and touch.

skull. The bony structure of the head consisting of the *cranium* and the *face.* The cranium is composed of eight bones, the face of fourteen.

sleeping sickness. *See* TRYPANOSOMIASIS.

slough (*sluff*). A mass of dead tissue separating from the surrounding living tissue, as in a wound.

smallpox. A serious, often fatal, contagious disease that comes on suddenly with high fever; in several days an eruption of small pimples appears all over the body. The eruption goes through a number of stages: increase in size of the pimple, blistering, pus formation, crusting, and pock marks. This whole procedure, if the patient lives, takes 12 to 14 days. Smallpox is caused by a virus and symptoms appear 12 to 21 days after the virus has entered the body of the susceptible individual.

smear. A preparation of blood, sputum, urine, or other body secretions for study under the microscope made by spreading on a glass slide.

smegma. Synonymous with sebum or the product of oil glands. —*s. clitoridis.* The material produced by the oil glands of the clitoris and the small vaginal lips. —*s. praeputii.* The substance produced by the oil glands of the foreskin.

snare. An instrument that has a wire loop that can be quickly narrowed by a mechanism in the handle, used to remove small growths that are attached by thin lengths of tissue, tonsils, and polyps.

sodomy. A form of sexual deviation, usually between males. 2. Bestiality.

soleus (*soh'lih-uhss*). A flat, broad muscle composing the part of the calf nearest the bone. *See* CALF.

soma. The entire body physically in distinction to the psyche.

somatic. 1. Pertaining to the body. 2. Relating to the body, excepting its organs, as the stomach, intestines, heart.

soporific. A sleep producer; narcotic.

sound. Air vibrations that are heard. —*breath sounds.* Sounds heard through the stethoscope upon the chest over the lungs, normal or diseased. —*fetal heart sounds.* The sounds produced by the heart of the developing infant in the womb; best heard near the mother's navel. —*heart sounds.* The heart when heard through a stethoscope has two sounds. The first is dull and long and sounds like *lub*, occurring at the same time the ventricles are squeezing out blood; the second is sharp and short and sounds like *dub*, occurring at the time the valves of the large arteries are closing to prevent leakage of blood back into the ventricle.

spasm. A sudden contraction of muscle.

spasticity. A state of sustained increased tension of a muscle.

specific. 1. A medication that has a special curative influence on a particular disease, as arsenic in syphilis and emetine in amoebic dysentery. 2. The specific disease produced by certain germs, as gonorrhea by the *Neisseria gonorrhea.* 3. Due to syphilis.

speculum (*spehk'yuh-luhm*). An instrument designed to increase the diameter of the opening of one of the body cavities in order more easily to visualize the inside, as a *nasal speculum, vaginal speculum.*

speech. Expressing thoughts by spoken words. *—ataxic s.* Speech that comes in explosive spurts through disorder of a certain part of the brain, the *cerebellum. —scanning s.* Speech in which there are pauses between the syllables in a certain definite rhythm, common in *multiple sclerosis. —slurred s.* Speech that is weak and trembling, characteristic of involvement of certain parts of the brain stem.

sperm. The fully developed germ cell of the male whose function is to penetrate a female egg cell to develop a new individual. Also called *spermatozoon.*

spermatocidal (*spuhr-maa-tuh-sigh'duhl*). Destructive of sperm, as the jellies used for contraception.

spermatozoa (*spuhr-maa-tuh-zoh'uh*). Plural of spermatozoon.

sphenoid. Wedge-shaped, as the bone that sits between the eyes behind the nose and that contains the sphenoid sinus.

sphenoiditis. Inflammation of the sphenoid sinus.

sphincter. A muscle that surrounds and closes an opening. *—anal s.* The muscles that surround the canal of the anus and close or open it.

sphygmograph (*sfihg'moh-graaf*). An instrument used to record by writing various characteristics of the pulse and blood pressure.

sphygmomanometer (*sfihg-moh-muh-nahm'ih-tuhr*). A blood-pressure machine.

spica (*spigh'kuh*). A bandage put on in spiral with reversed turns.

spina (*spigh'nuh*). A sharp protuberance. *—s. bifida.* A defect in development in which the spinal column is not closed, often with a protrusion of the covering of the spinal cord and at times nerve tissue. It most commonly occurs in the spine of the low back. *—s. bifida occulta.* A defect as above without the protrusion of the coverings of the spinal cord.

spine. 1. A sharp, thornlike piece of bone. 2. The spinal column or backbone.

spirochete (*spigh'ruh-keet*). Any one of a large group of spiral-shaped germs, as the syphilis germ.

splanchnic (*splaank'nihk*). Relating to, or supplying the internal organs, especially those within the abdominal cavity.

spleen. One of the organs of the abdominal cavity just below the diaphragm on the left side. The spleen is the largest lymph organ of the body and is covered by a tough, elastic sac of tissue that sends through it many small arms to form a large meshwork within the spleen. In the spaces of this meshwork there is red pulp arranged in cords and small spheres. The blood from all over the body eventually finds its way into and out of the spleen. The spleen functions as a storage place for red blood cells, feeding them to the blood stream as the body requires, and as the graveyard of red blood cells. In three to four weeks, the normal red cell grows old and is ready to be broken down. This breakdown occurs in the spleen where certain necessary elements within the blood cell, as iron, are extracted and stored. When severe bleeding occurs, the spleen forms new red cells and expresses them into the blood stream as replacements. It may also have a connection with the formation and storage of certain of the white blood cells.

splenectomy. The surgical removal of the spleen, performed as a curative measure in certain conditions, as purpura.

splenomegaly (*splehn-oh-mehg'uh-lih*). Enlargement of the spleen that occurs in a number of conditions, as leukemia, undulant fever, malaria, and certain types of hemolytic anemias.

splint. A piece of rigid material used to hold the ends of a broken bone together in an immovable position. Wood, metal, wire, plastic and hardened plaster are used. —*Thomas s.* A splint consisting of a ring that fits around the thigh or upper arm and two long metal rods that project from the ring on either side of the thigh or arm. The rods are joined by a crosspiece below the foot or hand, and this crosspiece is used for applying a measured pull on the lower fragment of the fractured bone. This splint is used not only to limit the movement of a broken arm and/or leg, but also to approximate the edges of the break by exerting a pull on the lower fragment of the fracture.

spondylalgia (*spahn-dih-laal'jih-uh*). Pain in a vertebra.

spondylitis. Inflammation of one or more vertebrae. —*ankylosing s.* Arthritis of the spine that includes involvement of the sacroiliac joints in the low back, the joints between the ribs and the spine when the thoracic region is involved, the ligaments that surround the spine, and at times the hips. Affects young men and is very disabling, producing a completely stiff back. It is called *bamboo spine, poker back, poker spine, rheumatoid arthritis of the spine, Marie-Strumpell disease*, and is also known by other names.

spot. A small area differing in appearance and/or activity from the area about it. —*genital s.* A small area in the lining tissue of the nose related to sex activity, particularly in the female. At times this area bleeds during menstruation. In the past, this area was coated with cocaine as treatment for painful menstruation. —*rose s.* An eruption of red pinhead elevations on the skin that fade when pressed. These occur most commonly on the abdomen and loins during the first week of typhoid fever.

sprain. Wrenching of a joint that causes a tear or stretching of the ligaments attached to the joint.

sprue. A disease of unknown cause, slow onset and long duration that is characterized by anemia, weakness, loss of weight, smooth reddish appearance of the tongue, and evacuation of unformed frothy stools in large amounts from the bowel. Most common in the East and West Indies, parts of Asia, but is also occasionally seen in the U. S.

spur. A pointed outgrowth, particularly of a bone. —*calcaneal s.* A painful, bony projection that grows out of the heelbone. Caused by injury, continuous standing, infections in other parts of the body, or improper shoes.

sputum (*spyou'tuhm*). A discharge from the lining tissue of the throat or mouth mostly expelled by spitting and at times by swallowing; composed of mucus, pus, saliva, alone or in any combination; often contains germs, blood, or any dusty material that is inhaled. —*purulent s*. Consists mostly of pus. —*rusty s*. Containing blood or deteriorated blood. Seen mostly in lobar pneumonia. Also called *prune juice s*.

squint. See STRABISMUS.

staff. Personnel of a hospital who are directly involved in caring for patients. —*consulting s*. Physicians who serve a hospital only in advisory capacity. —*house s*. The residents and interns living in a hospital. —*visiting s*. The physicians under whose direction the patients of a hospital are cared for.

stain. Used mostly to refer to a dye or pigment that has affinity for special parts of a structure or special cells, leaving others unaffected. Stains are used for the identification of bacteria under the microscope and also to make visible microscopic tissue structure that otherwise would be difficult or impossible to see, as *Wright's stain* for smears of blood, resulting in white blood cells showing up with either blue or red granules in their protoplasm, and the red cells in an orange or beige color.

stammering. Hesitant or interrupted speech.

stapes (*stay'peez*). One of the small bones of the middle ear shaped like a stirrup. The stapes is the innermost of the three small bones, the broad oval-shaped part of which attaches to the thin membrane covering an oval window in the internal ear.

Staphylococcus (*staaf-ih-loh-kahk'kuhss*). The general name of a spherical bacterium that, under the microscope, is seen to grow in clusters. There are many types of staphylococcus, a percentage of which produce disease with pus in man.

staphyloma. A bulging of the white or transparent part of the eye.

stasis (*stay'sihss*). A complete cessation of flow, as of the blood in a particular area or of the intestinal content.

status. A condition or state of being, often of extreme severity as *s. asthmaticus*, a state of asthma in which all of the symptoms are severely increased, difficult to relieve, long in duration, and at times fatal.

steatorrhea (*stee-uh-tuh-ree'uh*). 1. An excessive flow of oil from the oil glands. 2. Evacuated bowel contents containing undigested fat.

stenosis. Narrowing or reducing the diameter, particularly of an opening or a channel. —*aortic s.* In which the communication between the left chamber of the heart and the aorta is narrowed, usually due to disease of the valves here. —*mitral s.* Narrowing of the opening between the left atrium and the left large chamber of the heart, resulting from disease of the valve in this situation. Often an end result of rheumatic fever. —*pyloric s.* Obstruction of the communication between the lower end of the stomach and the first part of the small intestine, often present at birth due to an overdevelopment of the muscles in the wall of the lower end of the stomach.

stercolith. A dungstone. A concretion of feces that has hardened by the deposit of calcium salts.

stereoscope. An instrument that makes two somewhat overlapping pictures of the same object. When the pictures are viewed in the stereopticon they give the impression of depth.

sterility. The condition of inability to reproduce.

sterilization. 1. The process of destroying all forms of life, especially microscopic life, as germs and fungi. Heat, chemicals, ultraviolet light, are commonly used for sterilization. 2. Any method of making an individual incapable of reproduction. Surgery, as tying off the tubes in the female or the spermatic cord in the male; X-rays, intentional or unintentional, in the region of the ovaries or the testes; various diseases, particularly mumps, that affect the ovaries or testes.

sterilizer. An instrument used to destroy all forms of microscopic life. The commonest, the autoclave, uses steam under pressure at temperatures above the boiling point of water, much like the pressure cooker.

sternocleidomastoid (*stuhr-noh-kligh-doh-maas'toyd*). A muscle that is attached at its lower end to the top of the breastbone and the inner part of the collarbone, at its upper end to the mastoid bone just behind the ear. It functions in bending the head.

sternodynia. Pain in the breastbone. Also called *sternalgia*.

sternum. The breastbone. A flat, narrow bone in the middle of the front of the chest from the notch just below the neck to the point of the flare of the ribs, composed of three parts: a small upper portion, the *manubrium*; the major length, *the body*; and a small triangular tip, the *xiphoid*.

stertor. Snoring, or a snoring type of breathing; or the rattling sound when the voice box and the breathing tubes are filled with mucus.

stethoscope. An instrument used to detect sounds that arise within the body, having a cup, bell, or disc-shaped endpiece made of metal or hard rubber, that is connected to rubber tubing and conducts sound to both ears of the examiner.

stigma. Any one of the signs or marks that is characteristic of a condition. —*hysterical s.* Loss of sensation in the foot, leg, and lower part of the thigh, also called *stocking anesthesia*, characteristic of hysteria since the nerves of sensation in the leg are not distributed in this manner. Such loss of sensation therefore cannot be due to any true involvement of these nerves. There are many other symptoms of this condition that do not follow the pattern of physical disease. —*syphilitic s.* The signs of syphilis that are transmitted to the infant within the womb and are present on birth, as notched teeth, saber shins, deafness, and inflammation of the transparent part of the eye.

stimulant. Any agent or process that excites, stirs up, or increases activity.

stimulus. An irritant or exciting agent.

stomach. The most saclike part of the digestive tube, just below the diaphragm and somewhat to the left of center, shaped generally like a hand-scythe with a very wide blade.

At its upper or *cardiac end*, it is continuous with the gullet or esophagus; at its lower or *pyloric end*, with the first part of the small intestine or duodenum. Its wall is composed of four coats, an *inner mucous*, an *adjacent submucous*, a *muscular coat*, and a tough *outer lining*. The stomach produces gastric juice that contains hydrochloric acid and two special enzymes known as *pepsin* and *rennin*. Because of the arrangement of the muscles in the wall of the stomach that run longitudinally, obliquely, and circularly, the stomach actually churns the food that comes into it and mixes it with the gastric juice. Rennin curdles milk, changing the milk protein into casein. Pepsin acts on the proteins and begins the splitting up process. By virtue of another enzyme, *lipase*, fat is broken down to a small degree in the stomach.

stomatitis. Inflammation of the mouth due to germs that cause trench mouth, syphilis, tuberculosis; to fungi that cause thrush; to lack of vitamins, as vitamin C, that causes scurvy.

stool. The matter evacuated from the bowel. —*fatty s*. Stools in which there is fat, often caused by disease of the pancreas. —*tarry s*. Stools that look like tar, often the result of bleeding high up in the intestine or in the stomach. May be caused by medicine containing iron, barium, or bismuth.

strabismus. Squint. Cross-eye. —*conversion s*. Where the eye is crossed toward the nose. Also called *esotropia*. —*divergent s*. Where the squinting eye turns toward the temple. Also called *exotropia*.

strain. 1. A condition produced in a part by wrong use or overuse, as in eyestrain. 2. Undue stretching, as in muscle strain. 3. To make excessive effort.

strangulation. 1. Choking. 2. The clamping down on a part and cutting off the blood supply, as a hernia that is caught so tightly in the opening through which it protrudes that the blood supply is shut off from it. If not taken care of immediately, gangrene may develop.

Streptococcus. The name of a large tribe of germs, spherical bacteria, that under the microscope form chains, to which belong the germs causing gonorrhea, scarlet fever, rheumatic fever, and serious sore throats.

streptomycin. One of the newer antibiotics obtained from the mold *Streptomyces griseus.* It is effective against a host of germs, particularly those causing tuberculosis and tularemia. It may be given by injections under the skin, into the muscle, or into the spinal canal.

stria (*strigh'uh*). A narrow stripe or streak. —*s. albicans gravidarum.* The white, irregular streaks seen on the upper thighs and belly wall of pregnant women. —*s. atrophica.* White, irregular streaks of the skin seen where the skin has previously been stretched by injury, pregnancy, fat.

stricture. A narrowing of the passageway of a hollow organ or canal as of the gullet or urethra; the result of disease or injury in the surrounding walls. Stricture of the urethra or the passageway of urine through the penis was commonly due to gonorrhea before the newer antibiotic drugs appeared.

stridor (*strigh'duhr*). A harsh rasping sound produced on exhalation.

stroke. 1. A colloquial term for apoplexy. 2. A sudden seizure or fit of any disease.

Strongyloides (*strahn-gih-loy'deez*). A type of round worm. —*s. stercoralis.* Parasitic in the intestines of man; appears in the same areas as hookworm.

struma (*stroo'muh*). Goiter. —*Riedel's s.* Inflammation of the thyroid gland of long duration.

stupe. A cloth wrung out of hot water and sprinkled with turpentine or other counter-irritants used, in the past, to relieve intestinal bloating resulting from some diseases.

stupor. A state of insensibility or partial sensibility.

stutter. Speech with repeated efforts to speak a syllable.

stylet (*stigh'liht*). A wire that is inserted into a hollow needle to keep the opening clear or into a soft tube, as a catheter, to give it rigidity.

styptic (*stihp'tihk*). Any agent that stops bleeding by causing the blood vessels to close down, as the alum pencil used to check the bleeding of shaving cuts.

subacute. That stage of a disease after an initial height of symptoms and before the prolonged and perhaps continuous lower-grade symptoms.

subarachnoid (*sub-uh-raak′noyd*). Beneath the middle coat of tissue that lines the brain and spinal cord.

subclavian. Beneath the collarbone, as the *subclavian artery*.

subcutaneous. Under the skin; hypodermic.

sublimation. The turning of the stream of psychic energy from sexual aims to those nonsexual in nature and socially acceptable. Example: the pleasure a child takes in displaying himself nude, later transformed to the pleasure he takes in displaying his new clothes.

subluxation. A minor or incomplete slipping of a bone from its joint.

succussion. Shaking in order to determine whether or not fluid is present in a body cavity or hollow organ. —*s. sound*. The sound of splashing that is heard when the patient is shaken; may occur when there is air and fluid in the chest cavity or when the stomach is stretched and contains liquid.

sudamen (*syou-day′mehn*). A skin eruption of short duration that occurs after excessive sweating, consisting of whitish, almost transparent blisters caused by sweat collecting in the ducts of the sweat glands.

sudor. Sweat.

sudoresis (*syou-duh-ree′sihss*). Excessive sweating.

sudoriferous. Producing sweat.

suffusion. The spread or flow of any body liquid into surrounding tissue, often seen in severe injuries where a large collection of blood appears under a wide area of skin.

sulfa drugs. A group of drugs that have the property of preventing germs from increasing in numbers and reducing their activity. The most important are *sulfadiazine, sulfaguanidine, sulfanilamide, sulfathiazole*. Before the antibiotics, these drugs represented a marked advance in the treatment of certain infectious diseases, as gonorrhea, pneumonia, and streptococcus infection.

sunburn. Inflammation of the skin caused by the action of the sun's rays; discoloration of skin due to sun (tan).

sunstroke. A stroke resulting from exposure to the sun that results in a very high rise in temperature and may cause death if proper measures are not taken. The condition comes on not only because of high temperature but also because humidity interferes with the evaporation of perspiration.

superego. The conscience; the unconscious censor. A part of the psychological apparatus that arises early in life from the need to handle drives that are not permitted expression. The origin of the admonitions and commandments that the child hears from his parents or other sources is forgotten, as they gradually come to seem like an inner voice of hidden and supreme power, approving or disapproving all his actions and even thoughts. This becomes the superego.

superfecundation. When two or more egg cells are penetrated by sperm about the same period and during two or more successive acts of intercourse, not necessarily with the same male.

supernumerary. More than the usual number, as supernumerary breasts.

supinate (*soo'pih-nayt*). 1. To turn the arm so that the palm is up or faces front. 2. To turn the leg so that the sole is down or out. 3. To turn the body so that the chest and belly face up while lying down.

suppository. A medication made in varying shapes and weights of solid material for introduction into the various openings of the body. Ordinarily suppositories melt at body temperatures and in this way release medication. Examples: the rectal suppository for relief of the pain of piles; the vaginal suppository for contraception.

suppuration. The production of pus.

suspiration. A sigh.

susurration (*soo-suhr-ay'shuhn*). A murmur, as the sound of murmurs of the heart.

suture (*soo'chuhr*). 1. A line that represents the union between bones; a normal part of development, as the union of the bones of the skull. 2. A cordlike material that is used to sew up wounds, made of catgut, silk, fine metal. There are two major types of materials; those that are absorbed, as catgut; and those that are not absorbed and must be removed, as linen, silk, wire. There are many types of sutures classified according to the way they are placed in the tissue, as *continuous suture* that is similar to the technique of hemming a garment; *figure of eight* suture in which the suture is brought in and out of the tissues in the form of an 8.

sweat. The product of the sweat glands, consisting of a colorless, watery liquid that is composed of small amounts of fat, albumen, minerals, sugar, and other elements. By its evaporation from the skin it has a cooling effect and thus helps to regulate the body temperature.

sycosis. Any inflammation that involves the hair follicles, especially of the beard, characterized by tiny pimples with or without pus perforated by the hairs, and with crusting. —*s. parasitica, barber's itch.* A hair follicle disease due to the presence of fungi.

sympathectomy. A surgical removal of part of the sympaethetic nervous system; an operation for the treatment of certain types of high blood pressure.

symphysis (*sihm'fuh-sihss*). An immovable joint. —*s. mandibulae.* The vertical ridge that can be felt at the center of the chin and in some people is evident visually. It represents the union of the two halves of the lower jaw. —*s. pubis.* The union of the pubic bones just above the midline of the external genital.

symptom. The manifestation of disease as the patient experiences it. In contrast to *sign*, that is the manifestation of disease as the examiner perceives it. Headache is a symptom; rapid pulse is a sign.

syncope (*sihn'kuh-pee*). Fainting; a sudden loss of consciousness, usually resulting from lack of blood supply to the brain and may occur in heart conditions, spasms of the voice box, and other ailments.

syndactylus (*sihn-daak'tih-luhss*). A person with webbed fingers.

syndrome. A group of symptoms and signs that represent a specific type of injury or disease. The syndrome of asthma is cough, wheezing, difficulty in breathing.

synechia (*sih-nehk'ih-uh*). An abnormal union of parts, usually due to injury or disease. Particularly refers to the adherence of part of the iris to another part of the eye, as the cornea.

synovectomy. The surgical removal of the tissue that lines the interior of a joint.

synovitis. Inflammation of the lining membrane of a joint.

syphilid. Any skin eruption due to syphilis.

syphilis. A disease communicated by sexual contact, or innocently from blood or bite of infected person, or from infected mother to fetus; caused by a spiral bacterium known generally as a *spirochete*, specifically *Treponema pallidum*. Ordinarily the earliest manifestation of acquired syphilis is the *chancre* that usually appears on the genital but may appear on any part of the body, particularly the fingers, tongue, or tonsils. The chancre appears from ten days to three weeks after contact, is usually a painless ulcer, has a punched-out appearance with sharp edges, is moist, and may discharge pus. Shortly thereafter, the surrounding lymph glands swell and are known as *buboes*. This is *primary syphilis*. *Secondary syphilis* is characterized by ulcerations with an overgrowing whitish membrane on the lining tissues, eruptions of the skin, sore throat, enlargement of the lymph glands all over the body, and general symptoms of sickness. The third stage, known as *tertiary syphilis*, is characterized by an aggravation of the skin eruption that may become large ulcers and by a characteristic disorder known as the *gumma*, a mass of rubber-like consistency that may appear in any part or organ of the body. Between the secondary and tertiary stages there is a variable period of quiescence.

syringomyelia (*sih-rihn-goh-migh-ee′lih-uh*). A disease of unknown cause that produces cavities in the spinal cord near its center, resulting in characteristic types of sensation-loss. It is this condition in which people burn and injure themselves without knowing it.

system. 1. A combination of various parts into a whole, as the *respiratory system*, the *genitourinary system*. 2. The body as a whole.

systole (*sihs′tuh-lee*). The time during which the heart squeezes blood from the small chamber into the large chamber, or from the large chamber into the artery.

T

tabes (*tay′beez*). A shrinkage or wasting of tissues. Loosely used to mean a special type, *t. dorsalis.* —*diabetic t., diuretic t.* An involvement of nerves with a resulting shrinkage of muscles that the nerves supply, a condition of diabetes. —*spastic t.* A disease of the spinal cord that results in an inability to co-ordinate movements and spasm of the muscles of the legs. —*t. dolorosa.* A type in which pain is predominant. —*t. dorsalis.* Also known as *locomotor ataxia,* a disease caused by hardening of certain parts of the spinal cord resulting in sharp, shooting pains, unsteadiness, inability to co-ordinate movements, disorders of vision, loss of pain and touch sensation of the skin, severe episodes of girdlelike pain around the abdomen, the rectum, or the throat, a reduction of sex desire, a lack of control of the muscles of the anus, wasting of the joints often produced by syphilis. —*t. ergotica.* An end result of poisoning with ergot, the symptoms of which resemble *t. dorsalis.*

tabetic (*tuh-beht'ihk*). Relating to, or affected with, *tabes*, or *t. dorsalis.*

tachycardia (*taak-uh-kahr'dih-uh*). More rapid than normal heartbeat. Several varieties occur, described according to cause or to the site in the heart from which the unusually rapid stimulus of heart action originates. —*atrial t.* The stimulus arises in the muscle of the small chamber of the heart; the heart rate may be 160 to 200 a minute. —*atrio-ventricular t.* The stimulus arises in a small area between the large and small chambers of the heart; the rate varies between 100 and 270 per minute. —*paroxysmal t.* Fast beating of the heart that occurs in attacks. Between attacks the heart beats normally. —*ventricular t.* A beating of the large chamber of the heart at 150 to 250 per minute, independent of the regular beating of the small chamber.

tachypnea (*taak-ihp'nee-uh*). Unusually fast rate of breathing, not uncommonly occurs in hysteria or other emotional disturbances, at 40 breaths per minute (normal is 16-18).

tactile. Relating to the sense of touch.

Taenia (*tee'nih-uh*). The family name for a general type of worm, that is long, flat, sectional, much like a ribbon, ordinarily known as the tapeworm. —*t. echinococcus. See* ECHINOCOCCUS GRANULOSIS. —*t. saginata.* A tapeworm whose early stages are passed in cattle and adult stage in man's intestines. Humans acquire this infestation by eating insufficiently cooked infested beef. Also called *beef tapeworm.* —*t. solium.* Early stages of the tapeworm occur in hogs, later or adult stages in man's intestines. The infestation is ordinarily acquired by eating insufficiently cooked infested pork. Man may become a carrier of the young stage also. The young in this instance are called *cysticercus cellulosae.* Also called *pork tapeworm.*

talipes (*taa'luh-peez*). A general name for a variety of deformities of the foot, particularly those present from birth, as *clubfoot*. Talipes includes various deformities and simple distortions of the foot classified as to whether the foot is turned in or out and whether the Achilles' tendon that attaches the calf muscles to the heel bone is lengthened or shortened. —*t. calcaneus*. A type in which the individual walks on the heel bone. —*t. cavus*. A type in which the arch of the foot is markedly exaggerated. —*t. equinus*. A type in which the weight is borne upon the ball of the foot and the heel is elevated in walking. —*t. planus*. A type in which the arch of the foot is decreased or totally lost due to weakened ligaments. Also called *flatfoot*. —*t. valgus*. A type in which the outer border of the foot is raised and the ankle is turned inward with a flattened arch. Also called *pes planus, weak foot, flatfoot*. —*t. varus*. A type in which the outer border of the foot is turned down, most of the weight being borne here. When this down turning is extreme and the foot is turned inward the condition is known as *clubfoot*.

talus. The uppermost anklebone upon which the bones of the leg rest. Formerly called *astragalus*.

tampon. A plug, usually of cotton or other material, inserted into a cavity, as the vagina or the nose, for application of medicine or exertion of pressure in order to stop bleeding.

tamponade. The act of plugging. —*cardiac t*. A serious condition in which a large amount of fluid accumulates in the sac around the heart, causing a marked embarrassment of heart action. Unless cared for by drainage, death may result.

tapeworm. Any of the large class of long, flat, segmented, ribbon-like worms that are parasites on man and other animals. —*beef t. Taenia saginata*. —*broad t*. or *fish t. Diphyllobothrium latum*. —*dog t. Dipylidium caninum*. —*dwarf t. Hymenolepis nana*. —*mouse t. Hymenolepis diminuta*. —*pork t. Taenia solium*.

tarsitis (*tahr-sigh'tihss*). Inflammation of the gristle in the eyelid.

tarsus. 1. The ankle or instep, composed of six bones. 2. The thick, tough, supporting tissue that gives the eyelid its firmness.

telangiectasis (*teh-laan-jih-ehk'tuh-sihss*). A state of marked widening of groups of minute blood vessels, the capillaries. These form dark red, wartlike spots that vary in size from a pinhead to a pea.

temple. The part of the head above the cheekbones and behind the eye.

temporal. 1. Relating to the temple, as the temporal bone. 2. Relating to time.

tenderness. A condition of unusually great sensitivity to touch; soreness.

tendon. A band of tough, fibrous tissue that attaches muscle to bone.

tenesmus (*tuh-nehz'muhss*). A painful, unsuccessful straining to empty the bowels or the urinary bladder, occurring in certain stages of intestinal or bladder inflammation.

tennis arm. Tennis elbow. An inflammation of the lining membrane of the elbow joint common in tennis players. Also called *radio-humeral bursitis.*

tenonitis. An inflammation of the sheath about a tendon.

tenonometer (*tehn-uh-nahm'ih-tuhr*). An instrument that is placed upon the eyeball to measure the pressure within it.

tenoplasty. Surgical repair of a tendon.

tenosynovitis (*tehn-uh-sihn-uh-vigh'tihss*). Inflammation of a tendon and its sheath.

tenotomy (*teh-naht'uh-mih*). The surgical cutting of a tendon.

tension. The state of being strained or stretched. —*arterial t.* The strain in the walls of an artery when it is filled by a new gush of blood from the area above or from the heart. —*premenstrual t.* Unusually marked nervous and circulatory symptoms present in menstruation, severe and long-lasting enough to require treatment. Examples are emotional breakdown with weeping, nervousness, lack of concentration, and headache.

teratology. The science that deals with monstrosities and malformations.

teratoma (*tehr-uh-toh'muh*). A tumor that contains hair, teeth, or other materials not found in the area where the tumor grows. Teratoma is the result of a misplacement of tissue during development of the infant within the womb.

test. 1. An examination. 2. A method of identifying a contained material, or changes in the activity of organs or systems, or of determining the true nature of a condition. —*Ascheim-Zondeck, A-Z t.* Injection into white mice of urine from a woman. If the woman is pregnant, the ovaries of the mice enlarge, fill with blood, and the egg cells develop and make ready for discharge. —*Benedict's t.* A test used by diabetics to determine the presence of sugar in the urine. Eight drops of urine are added to five c.c. of a special solution and boiled for three minutes. If the normal blue of the solution is unchanged, no sugar is present; if a green, yellow, or red sediment appears sugar is present. —*brucellergin t.* A test made to determine the presence of undulant fever. An extract of undulant fever germs is injected into the skin. The appearance of an elevated red area at the injection site indicates the presence of the germ in the body, at the time the test is made or in the past. —*cold pressor t.* The blood pressure of an individual is taken. Then one hand is immersed in ice water for one minute and the blood pressure taken again. Those who show an unusual rise in blood pressure or whose blood pressure returns to normal slowly are considered likely to develop high blood pressure. —*Dick t.* A test for susceptibility or immunity to scarlet fever. A small amount of specially prepared bacterial culture of the streptococcus that is responsible for scarlet fever is injected into the skin. If within 24 hours a redness and elevation appears in this area, it indicates susceptibility to scarlet fever; if a redness is not present, immunity to scarlet fever is indicated. —*erythrocyte sedimentation t.* Blood is drawn from a vein and a citrate or oxalate solution is added to prevent clotting. The blood is drawn into a narrow tube and permitted to stand. Normally, the red blood cells will settle to the bottom. The rate of this settling is the test and indicates the presence of various conditions. —*Friedman t.* A test of pregnancy by injecting urine of a patient thought to be pregnant into the vein of a female rabbit. If the woman is pregnant the ovaries of the rabbit will show red, blood-filled masses on their surface. —*frog t.* Another test for pregnancy. The urine of a pregnant woman is injected into a female African frog. Within 12 hours 5 or more eggs will be deposited. —*glucose tolerance t.* This test is aimed at determining the ability of the liver to transform the free sugar as it exists in the blood (glucose) into stored sugar as it exists in the liver (glycogen). The test is performed by giving the patient a specific amount of glucose (either by vein or mouth) on a fasting stomach. At regular intervals thereafter, blood is drawn and the level of glucose is determined in each specimen. These findings are plotted on a graph, and the resulting curve indicates the status of this function of the liver. Especially important to determine the severity of diabetes mellitus and the presence of other conditions. —*histamine t.* 1. The injection of histamine beneath the skin induces the stomach to produce hydrochloric acid. Histamine injection determines whether or not the stomach is capable of producing hydrochloric acid. Important in such conditions as *pernicious anemia.* 2. Injection of histamine to determine whether or not it is responsible for a certain type of headache from which the patient suffers. —*Ishihara's t.* A test of color vision made by using a number of plates upon which are printed dots of various sizes and colors. —*Kahn t.* A test for syphilis performed on blood serum. —*Klein t.* A test for syphilis performed on blood serum. —*Kolmer's t.* A test for syphilis using red blood cells. —*Mantoux t.* A test for tuberculosis in which protein of the germs of tuberculosis is injected into the skin. If the patient has or has had tuberculosis, swelling, redness, and even ulceration may appear at the test site within 48 hours. —*Mazzini t.* A test for syphilis made on the blood serum. *—occult blood t.* A test made on material evacuated from the bowel to determine the presence of blood. *—Papanicolau t.* A test for cancer of the neck of the womb. Performed by examining the discharge of the vagina under the microscope for abnormal cells. *—Schick t.* A test to determine immunity to diphtheria. A small amount of toxin from diphtheria germs is injected into the skin. Within 5 to 7 days there is swelling and redness at the site of injection if the patient is susceptible to diphtheria. *—Schiller t.* A test for cancer based on the fact that cancerous tissue does not stain mahogany-brown with an iodine solution. *—syphilis t.* There are more than a dozen of these, each with its advantages. *—Wassermann's t.* A test for syphilis.

testis. The male reproductive gland which, when mature, is the source of sperm. *—abdominal t.* A testis that has not followed the normal pattern of development from the abdomen into the groin and then into the scrotum, but has remained in the abdomen. *—inguinal t.* A testis that has not descended into the scrotum but that has remained in its course of descent in the groin. *—undescended t.* The condition in which a testis has not descended into its normal position in the scrotum.

testosterone (*tess-tahss'tuh-rohn*). One of the hormones produced by the testes that controls the male secondary sex characteristics, such as hair and fat distribution, timbre of voice. Also made synthetically. Commonly called the male hormone.

tetanus. 1. An infectious disease caused by the poison produced by the tetanus germ, *Clostridium tetani*, that enters the body through a wound. This poison stimulates a constant spasm of the muscles under the control of the will, and severe convulsions. The most dangerous kind of wounds are puncture wounds, penetrating wounds, and crushing injury. It is commonly called *lockjaw.* 2. A state of spasm of a muscle.

tetany. A disease that is characterized by episodes of painful spasms of the muscles with convulsive movements, usually due to a lack of, or an inability to utilize, calcium. Tetany occurs where the parathyroid glands are not producing enough hormones; where there is an abnormal amount of bicarbonate in the blood stream; where the vitamin-D intake is insufficient; and where the parathyroid glands have been removed by surgery. —*hyperventilation t.* A form due to forced breathing, usually in cases of emotional disturbance where the carbon dioxide is washed out of the blood stream with a resulting relative increase in the bicarbonate.

thalamus (*thaal'uh-muhss*). A most important part of the brain, situated at its base, that serves as a relay station for impulses to and from the brain relating to higher mental and emotional activity; loosely called the seat of the emotions.

thelerethism (*thih-lehr'uh-thihsm*). Erection of the nipple.

thelitis (*thih-ligh'tihss*). Inflammation of the nipple.

thelium. The nipple.

thenar (*thee'nahr*). 1. The palm. 2. The fleshy mound on the palm just below the thumb. 3. Relating to the palm, as the thenar muscles.

therapeusis (*thehr-uh-pyou'sihss*). A branch of medical science that deals with the treatment of disease. Also called *therapeutics*.

therapy. Treatment. —*collapse t.* Treatment of tuberculosis of the lung that aims at decreasing the volume of the lung in order to rest it and close any cavities within the compressed part. Many procedures are used for this purpose, as the introduction of air into the chest cavity, removal of several or all of the ribs on one or both sides, or paralyzing the diaphragm by interrupting its nerve, the *phrenic nerve*. —*glandular t.* The treatment of diseases by extracts made from glands or organs that furnish hormones necessary for the body. —*intravenous t.* The use of curative materials introduced into the veins. —*maggot t.* The treatment of infection of the bone marrow and bone by the use of the maggot of the bluebottle fly. Introduced into the wound, it eats the decayed material. —*malarial t.* Artificially producing malaria in a patient with syphilis of the nervous system. Beneficial because of the repeated attacks of fever. —*occupational t.* Used mostly in patients with emotional and mental diseases, inducing them to pursue hobbies or trades. —*physical t.* The treatment of disease by various physical agents, as heat, cold, massage, light. —*radium t.* The use of radium to destroy tissues, usually cancerous. —*shock t.* Therapy used for treatment of psychotic disorders such as schizophrenia by administering certain drugs or electric shocks which produce coma and convulsions. *See also* PSYCHOTHERAPY.

thoracectomy (*thaw-ruh-sehk'tuh-mih*). The surgical removal of a rib.

thoracentesis (*thaw-ruh-sehn-tee'sihss*). The introduction of a needle between the ribs into the chest cavity in order to remove fluid.

thoracoplasty. 1. The operation in which any number of ribs, entire or in part, are removed in order to collapse the chest wall. 2. Cutting adhesions between the diseased lung and the chest wall.

thorax. The chest. The part of the trunk below the neck and above the diaphragm. Within the chest are contained the heart and its sac, the lungs and their coverings, the large vessels, part of the gullet, the bronchi, and the major lymph duct.

thrill. A fine vibration that can be felt over certain diseased arteries, a heart with diseased valves, and certain types of cysts.

thrombin. A substance in the blood through the action of which clotting takes place.

thrombinogen (*thrahm-bihn'oh-jehn*). An element in the fluid part of the blood that is an early stage in the development of thrombin. Also called *prothrombin, thrombogen, serozyme,* and *proserozyme.*

thromboangiitis (*thrahm-boh-aan-jih-igh'tihss*). Inflammation of the inner coat of a blood vessel with the presence of a blood clot. —*t. obliterans.* A disease with widespread inflammation of veins and accumulation of tough, fibrous tissue around the arteries and nerves that accompany these veins.

Because it results in a cutoff of blood supply, gangrene of a part necessitating amputation is common. Seems to affect young to middle-aged males chiefly. Also called *Buerger's disease*.

thrombocyte. A colorless, small disc that is important in the clotting of blood. *See* PLATELET.

thrombocytopenia (*thrahm-boh-sigh-toh-pee'nih-uh*). A decrease in the number of thrombocytes or blood platelets; seen in various bleeding diseases, as *purpura*.

thrombophlebitis (*thrahm-boh-flih-bigh'tihss*). The inflammation of a vein associated with clotting of blood.

thrombosis. The formation of a blood clot.

thrombus. A blood clot that is formed in the blood vessels or the heart, due ordinarily to a change in the character of the blood or in the walls of the blood vessels, or to a slowing of circulation of the blood.

thrush. An infestation with a yeastlike germ, *Candida albicans*. Thrush is a disease of children in which the tip and sides of the tongue and the mucous membrane lining the cheeks are covered with small, whitish spots.

thumb. The finger on the inner side of the hand that differs from other fingers in that it is composed of only two bones, and that the long bone of the hand to which it is attached is freely movable.

thymus (*thigh'muhss*). A gland that is situated upon the windpipe, develops until the second year, remains stationary until the fourteenth, and then gradually shrinks away.

thyroid. Literally means shield-shaped. Actually the thyroid is in the shape of a squat H, the two vertical bars somewhat wide and oval, the horizontal bar small. Situated in the front of the neck, it secretes a hormone known as *thyroxin*, which is vital to life.

thyroidectomy. The surgical removal of part or all of the thyroid gland.

thyroiditis. Inflammation of the thyroid gland.

thyrotoxicosis. A condition of excess activity of the thyroid gland regardless of cause.

thyroxin. The hormone produced by the thyroid gland.

tibia (*tihb'ih-uh*). The shinbone; the larger of the two bones of the leg that composes part of the knee-joint above and the ankle-joint below.

tic. A twitching of a muscle, especially of the muscles of the face. —*t. douloureux.* Attacks of severe pain in the face described by some as the most severe pain that can be experienced.

time. The duration of an event or a manifestation. —*bleeding t.* The time it takes for the bleeding due to the puncture of a finger tip or an earlobe to stop. Normally one to three minutes. —*clot retraction t.* The time it takes for a clot to form and shrink in freshly drawn blood. Usually one hour. —*clotting t.* The time it takes for a clot to form in freshly drawn blood. Ordinarily five to eight minutes.

timothy. The common name for an important fodder grass in America. It pollinates from the middle of May to the middle of July and is one of the most common causes of summer hay fever. It is named after Timothy Hanson, who introduced the seed to Carolina about 1720.

tinea (*tihn'ih-uh*). The skin manifestation produced by certain molds; ringworm. —*t. barbae.* Ringworm of the face and neck. Also called *barber's itch* and *t. sycosis.* —*t. capitis.* A fungus infection of the scalp and hair. Also called *t. tonsurans.* —*t. corporis.* A fungus infection of the skin of the trunk. —*t. cruris.* A fungus infection of the groin, the area around the anus, the area between the anus and genital. —*t. pedis.* A fungus infection of the feet, particularly between the toes. Also called *athlete's foot.* —*t. ungulum.* A fungus infection of the toe and fingernails. —*t. versicolor.* A fungus infection of the trunk.

tinnitus (*tih-nigh'tuhss*). A ringing, hissing, or roaring sound in the ears.

tissue. A collection of cells of the same type and the substance that holds them together. *—adipose t.* Made up essentially of fat that is arranged in a loose meshwork of supporting tissue. *—connective t.* A general term for the various supporting tissues of the body whose function is to hold together the specialized functioning cells. Among these are adipose tissue, bone, gristle, tough, fibrous tissue, and others. *—erectile t.* A tissue much like a sponge consisting of spaces containing blood that, when their blood content is increased, enlarge and become firm, as in the penis and clitoris. *—fibrous connective t.* The strongest, densest supporting tissue of the body, the substance of tendons, ligaments, and coverings of the nervous system. *—glandular t.* A group of cells whose function is to manufacture secretions.

toe. A digit of the foot. *—hammer t.* See HAMMERTOE. *—Morton's t.* See METATARSALGIA.

tolerance. The ability to withstand the effect of a drug or a poison, especially when this ability is acquired or enhanced by continual use of the substance. *—sugar t.* The tolerance of a diabetic for sugar that is measured in a special way by determining the maximum amount of sugar he can take that does not cause sugar to appear in the urine.

tongue. The movable organ, made largely of muscle, attached to the floor of the mouth and involved in speaking, tasting, chewing, and swallowing. The muscles of this organ are covered by a moist membrane that has numerous elevations within which are found the *taste buds*.

tonsil. A mass of lymph tissue found in the throat as a pair, one on either side of the back of the mouth, in special niches known as *tonsillar fauces*. *—lingual t.* Tonsil tissue found on the back of the tongue. *—palatine t.* Technical term for tonsils. *—pharyngeal t.* A tonsil found on the back wall of the throat behind the nose, prominent in childhood, and commonly called *adenoids*.

tonsillectomy. Removal of the tonsils.

tonsillitis. Inflammation of the tonsils.

tophus (*toh'fuhss*). A chalky deposit found about the joints and in the external ear, especially in gout.

torticollis (*tor-tih-kahl'lihss*). A painful spasm of the muscles in the neck that run from the region just behind the ear to the top of the breastbone and collarbone, causing the head to be bent forward and to one side. Also called *wryneck*.

tourniquet (*tuhr'nih-keht*). Any material that can be used to exert pressure on a part in order to control bleeding or circulation. Made in many forms from a necktie, rope, or handkerchief that is tightened with a stick in an emergency, to straps, rubber tubes, cords, or other more elaborate instruments.

toxemia. A condition in which poison, produced by cells of the body or by the growth of a germ, is found in the blood. Usually when the blood contains poison produced by germs but not germs themselves, a state of general infection exists.

toxicity (*tahk-sihs'ih-tih*). The quality of being poisonous.

toxicology. The science that deals with poisons, their nature, results, detection, and treatment.

toxin. The poisonous product of animal or vegetable cells that, when gaining access into man or animal, stimulates the production of a specific protective substance against itself known as antitoxin. The most important toxins are those produced by germs. Those produced by plants are called *phytotoxins*, as *ricin* from the castor bean, and *abrin* from the seed of the Indian licorice. Those produced by animals, *zootoxins*, are snake venoms and spider poison.

toxoid. A toxin treated so that its poisonous quality is removed, but its quality of causing the production of protective antitoxin still remains. Used commonly in immunization against diphtheria and tetanus.

trachea (*tray'kih-uh*). The windpipe; extends from the lower end of the voice box into the chest where it divides into the major breathing tubes or bronchi.

tracheitis (*tray-kih-igh'tihss*). Inflammation of the windpipe.

tracheotomy. The surgical cutting into the trachea, usually performed as a lifesaving measure where the windpipe is blocked and air cannot get into the lungs. By making an incision below the blockage, breathing can take place through the new opening, instead of through the nose and mouth.

trachoma (*truh-koh'muh*). A communicable disease of the eyelids due to a virus producing small, blister-like elevations on the lining tissue of the lid that later scar over, contract, and cause deformity of the lid. The constant friction of these elevations may cause ulcerations or an overgrowth with blood vessels in the transparent part of the eye and may result in blindness.

traction. Drawing or pulling; as the pull maintained with weights and pulleys on a fragment of bone that has been broken in order to keep the ends of the broken bone head-on, so that healing can take place in the proper position.

transference. The displacement of feeling or emotion one associates with one person or idea to another. This occurs particularly during psychoanalysis when the patient unconsciously attaches to the person of the analyst the feelings and emotions the patient had toward parents during infancy. This results in feelings of love or hate for the analyst which have no basis in fact. Since these arise from the unconscious, the patient has no understanding as to why he feels the way he does about the analyst.

transfusion. Ordinarily used to mean a transfer of blood into a vein. There are many methods, generally divided into the *indirect*, where blood from the donor is collected in a bottle and mixed with a clotting preventative such as sodium citrate and then introduced into the vein of the recipient; and the *direct* or *immediate*, where the transfer of blood from one person to another is direct without the use of a clotting preventative and is usually done by syringe.

transillumination. Usually used to mean the lighting up of the sinuses about the nose by means of a light placed in the patient's mouth. Often shows the presence of abnormal material within the sinuses or distortion of the walls. May be used to light up other parts or cavities.

transplant. The tissue that is removed from any part of the body and placed on another area, as skin from the thigh applied to a denuded part of the arm.

transvestitism. The uncontrollable desire to dress in the clothing of the opposite sex.

trapezius (*traa-pee'zih-uhss*). A large muscle that arises from the base of the skull, the spine of the neck, and the spine of the thorax and attaches to the collarbone, the shoulder, and an extension of the shoulder blade, acting to raise the shoulder and draw the shoulder blade backward.

trauma (*traw'muh*). An injury or a wound; used in psychiatry to mean a severe emotional injury that leaves a deep impression.

tremor. A trembling, usually in rhythmic movement, of part of or an entire voluntary muscle. —*intention t.* A slow, coarse trembling of the limbs, exaggerated when motion is attempted. The trembling may disappear on rest and is very common in certain diseases of the nervous system, especially *multiple sclerosis.* —*pill-rolling t.* A description of the behavior of the hand in shaking palsy. The thumb and forefinger move against one another as though a pill were being rolled between them.

trench foot. A condition of the feet in those exposed in the trenches. Resembles frostbite.

trephine (*trih-fighn'*). A circular instrument with saw edges used for cutting out a button of bone, especially from the skull.

trephining. The operation of removing a button of bone with a trephine; also used to mean the removal of a part of the outer coat of the eyeball to relieve the pressure within the eyeball in *glaucoma.*

Treponema (*trehp-oh-nee'muh*). A class of bacteria that are spiral in form. —*t. pallidum.* The germ that causes syphilis. —*t. pertenue.* The germ that causes yaws.

triad. A group of three symptoms, objects, or elements. *—Hutchinson's t.* A combination of inflammation of the cornea, notched teeth, and deafness; found in people who have syphilis from birth.

trichiasis (*trih-kigh'uh-sihss*). The turning in of the eyelashes due to their abnormal position, causing irritation of the eyeball by friction. May be an inherited condition, or follow an inflammation of the lid with distortion.

trichinella. A type of worm that is a parasite in many animals, such as the cat, dog, rat, pig, and man. *—t. spiralis.* The type of trichinella that is a parasite in man.

trichinosis (*trihk-ih-noh'sihss*). Infestation with *t. spiralis* due to eating infested pork. The symptoms are fever, nausea, diarrhea, dizziness, prostration, stiffness and pain in the muscles, and swelling of the face.

trichitis. Inflammation of the hair roots.

trichology (*trih-kahl'uh-jee*). The study of the hair and its diseases.

trichomonas. The name of a large group of microscopic one-celled animals that have from three to five whip-like appendages (*flagellae*) to propel them. *—t. hominis.* A type found in the intestine of man. Not disease-producing. *—t. vaginalis.* A type found in the vagina that may cause inflammation.

Trichophyton. A general name for a large group of fungi that attach themselves to the nails, skin, and hair, often responsible for allergic reactions.

trichophytosis (*trihk-oh-figh-toh'sihss*). A contagious disease of the skin and hair, occurring most in children, due to the trichophyton fungus. Circular, scaly patches and partial loss of hair are the common symptoms.

triorchid (*trigh-awr'kihd*). Having three testes.

triquetrum (*trigh-kwee'truhm*). One of the bones of the wrist. Formerly called *cuneiform*.

trismus (*trihz'muhss*). A spasm of the muscles of chewing.

trocar. A surgical instrument used to puncture cavities for the removal of the contained fluid. To all effects a large-sized needle as used on a syringe. Consists of a rigid, hollow tube into which is introduced a snug-fitting, pointed rod that extends just beyond the end of the tube. Fitted together, it is used as a puncturing instrument. When in the cavity, the rod is removed to permit the fluid to flow freely through the tube.

trochanter (*troh-kaan'tuhr*). The name of two extensions of bone from the upper part of the thighbone. The *greater t.* is on the outside and can be felt just under the hip-joint; the *lesser t.* is on the inside.

trunk. 1. The body without head or limbs; the torso. 2. The main portion of a nerve, blood, or lymph vessel.

Trypanosoma (*trihp-uh-nuh-soh'muh*). A type of microscopic one-celled animal with a single whiplike projection that helps in its movement. It is transmitted to man by insects. —*t. gambiense*. The organism causing mid-African sleeping sickness. —*t. rhodesiense*. The organism causing East African sleeping sickness.

trypanosomiasis (*trihp-uh-nuh-soh-migh'uh-sihss*). Any of the diseases due to infection with trypanosoma, characterized by irregular fever and enlarged lymph glands.

tsetse fly (*tseht'see*). A fly almost entirely restricted to Africa that carries the *trypanosoma*, transmitting it to animal and man.

tsutsugamushi disease. A disease characterized by headache, fever and rash caused by a germ, *Rickettsia tsutsugamushi*, transmitted to man by the bite of the young forms of an insect, *trombicula*. Occurs particularly in the South Pacific Islands, Japan, and Formosa. Also called *Japanese river fever*, *Sumatran mite typhus, scrub typhus, Malayan typhus*, and *Queensland coastal fever*.

tubercle (*too'buhr-kuhl*). 1. A small swelling. 2. A rounded elevation on a bone. 3. The specific change in tissue caused by the tuberculosis germ.

tubercular. Characterized by the presence of tubercles or small swellings. Often used incorrectly, in place of tuberculous, to mean infected with tuberculosis.

tuberculin. A material made from the tuberculosis germ that contains its protein fraction, capable of causing inflammation in tissues of a human or animal who has or has had tuberculosis. Tuberculin is used as a skin test. A small amount is injected into the skin. Within 48 hours an elevation, redness, and at times an ulceration will result in people who have become allergic to the germ of tuberculosis. Such a reaction indicates past or present infection with tuberculosis.

tuberculosis. An infectious disease caused by the tubercle bacillus known as the *Myobacterium tuberculosis*. Although tuberculosis may affect any part of the body, the most common area of involvement is the lungs. —*minimal t.* Tuberculosis of the lung in which there are no cavities and in which the amount of lung tissue involved is very small. —*moderately advanced t.* Tuberculosis in which lung tissue equivalent to one lung is involved and in which the large areas of involvement do not affect more than the equivalent of one-third of a lung. The total diameter of the cavity or cavities must not exceed one and a half inches. —*open t.* Tuberculosis of the lung in a stage in which it is capable of transmission to other people. —*primary t.* The body reaction against the first intrusion of tuberculosis germs. Always heals over with calcification and is frequently overlooked or considered a condition not worthy of attention. Occurs usually early in life. Since it often appears in the lungs, casual X-rays of the lungs frequently show a small healed-over area in the lung tissue and some enlargement of the lymph glands near the large breathing tubes.

tuberculous. Caused by or having tuberculosis.

tuberosity (*too-buh-rahs'uh-tih*). A projection on a bone.

tularemia (*too-luh-ree'mih-uh*). A disease caused by a germ known as *Pasteurella tularensis* that is transmitted to man by handling infected rabbits or other rodents, or by the bite of a blood-sucking insect.

tumescence. A swelling.

tumor. A new growth of cells or tissue, of unknown cause, that is independent of the laws of growth of the individual upon which it arises. It may kill its host. There are many types of tumors classified according to the tissue from which they arise and whether or not they are a serious threat to life.

turbinate. A scroll-shaped, irregular bone on the side wall of the nose composed of an upper, middle, and lower part through which run the openings of several of the nasal sinuses.

turgor (*tuhr'guhr*). Swelling; the presence of an undue amount of blood within the small blood vessels in a part.

tussis. A cough. —*t. convulsiva.* Whooping cough.

twin. One of two individuals of the same birth. —*fraternal twins.* Twins that are the result of fertilization of two separate egg cells. May be entirely different individuals in sex, looks, stature, mentality. —*identical twins.* Twins that develop from a single fertilized egg cell. Are always of the same sex, stature, mentality.

tympanites (*tihm-puh-nigh'teez*). A tense protrusion of the abdominal wall due to bloating or accumulation of gas in the intestinal tract or the abdominal cavity.

typhoid. An acute infectious disease caused by an organism, *Eberthella typhosa*, that enters the body in food and water, and is found in the intestines and in the bowel discharge. The spleen and the lymph glands surrounding the intestines are enlarged and the lining membrane of the intestines is inflamed. Two or three weeks after the germ has entered the body, the disease sets in with headache, pains and aches, nosebleed, and diarrhea. The temperature rises gradually each evening and reaches 105°, at which level it remains for several weeks and gradually disappears. The tongue eventually becomes dry and brown. There is complete loss of appetite; the bowels are loose; there is often a mild cough and congestion of the lungs. After a week, a rose-colored eruption appears, particularly on the abdomen and chest. Many nerve symptoms occur, as deafness, stupor, delirium. Important complications are bleeding from the intestines; perforation of the intestines with resulting peritonitis; pneumonia; and inflammation of the kidneys. Second attacks are very rare.

typhus. An infectious disease with a sudden onset, transmitted to man by the body louse and the rat flea infected with an organism, the *Rickettsea prowazekii*. The first symptoms are severe pain in the back, limbs, and head; a rapidly rising fever from 104° to 105°. On the fourth or fifth day, an eruption of rose-colored spots appears all over the body, shortly becoming bloody. The complications are pneumonia, and inflammation of the kidneys. Also called *jail fever, ship fever, camp fever. —scrub t.* Another name for *Tsutsugamushi disease.*

U

ulcer. An excavated sore, the base of which is inflamed. —*decubitus u.* A bedsore. An ulceration of the skin and the tissue beneath the skin due to long pressure against the bed. Seen particularly in the aged, but may occur if care is not taken frequently to move a patient confined to bed for a long time. —*duodenal u.* An ulcer in the *duodenum* or first part of the small intestine, usually on the inner surface of its front wall near the *pylorus* or lower end of the stomach. Also called *peptic u.* —*gastric u.* An ulcer of the lining tissue of the stomach. —*marginal u.* An ulcer of the *jejunum,* or second part of the small intestine, near the mouth of a surgically made communication between the stomach and this part of the intestine. The surgical procedure that makes this communication is called a *gastroenterostomy* and is performed to short-circuit food around an existing ulcer in the lower end of the stomach or the upper end of the small intestine. Marginal ulcer is believed to be due to the destructive action of the acid in the gastric juice upon the lining tissue of the jejunum. —*peptic u.* An ulcer due to the destructive action of acid gastric juice upon the lining tissue of the stomach, duodenum, or jejunum. —*perforating u.* The ulcer that extends through the entire wall of an organ. —*rodent u.* An ulcer due to a certain type of cancer called *basal-cell carcinoma* that penetrates deeply from the skin and affects particularly the face, neck, and scalp. It is ordinarily remedied by surgery and is only mildly threatening to life. —*tropical u.* A skin ulcer common in the tropics.

ulceration. The formation of an ulcer.

ulna. The bone on the inner side of the forearm that with the lower end of the arm bone makes up the elbow joint.

ultrafiltration. The passage of liquid material through a filter that has very minute pores, such as clay, porcelain, or very thick and specially prepared filter paper. Ordinarily this process is performed with the aid of pressure or suction. Its purpose is to remove the very finest particles from the liquid. Usually by such filtration particles as small as the ordinary germ, but not as small as the viruses, can be removed.

umbilicus (*uhm-bihl'ih-kuhss*). The navel. The round depression in the low center of the abdomen, the scar of the site where the cord of the afterbirth was implanted in the individual during his development in the womb. Also called the *belly button.*

uncinate fits (*uhn'suh-nayt*). Attacks of hallucinations of smell associated with a dreamy state and smacking movements of the lips, the result of disturbance in the area of the brain that controls the sense of smell.

unconscious. The area below the level of awareness where exist multiple emotional and mental processes such as conflicts, complexes and their opposing forces, pushed into this area by repression and maintained there by resistance. It is from the various interactions of these forces in the unconscious that emotional and mental symptoms arise.

underweight. A condition of general deficiency of tissue, particularly fat, in the whole body. Usually applied to those whose weight is 10 per cent or more below that of average persons of the same height, sex, and age.

undulant fever. *See* BRUCELLOSIS.

unguis (*un'goo-ihss*). A finger or toenail. —*u. incarnatus.* Ingrowing nail.

unilateral. Relating to, or involving, only one side.

union. A juncture; particularly refers to the joining together of breaks in the bone.

ureter (*you-ree'tuhr*). A long, slender tube that is the passageway for urine from the pelvis of the kidney to the bladder.

ureterolith. A stone in the ureter.

ureterotomy. A surgical incision of the ureter.

urethra (*you-ree'thruh*). The passageway of urine from the bladder to the outside. In the male it is about 8 to 9 inches long and serves also to convey sperm. It is divided into three sections: the *prostatic portion,* which is within the prostate gland; the *membranous portion,* which is between the prostate and the penis; and the *spongy* or *penile portion* that is within the penis. In the female, it is about one and a half inches long.

urethritis (*you-ruh-thrigh'tihss*). Inflammation of the urethra. —*anterior u.* Inflammation of that part of the urethra that is within the penis. —*posterior u.* Inflammation of the urethra between the bladder and penis. —*simple u.* Inflammation of the urethra not due to gonorrhea. —*specific u.* Inflammation of the urethra as a result of gonorrhea.

urgency. A compelling desire to empty the bladder or the bowel.

urine. The liquid excreted by the kidneys, normally amber in color with a faint odor, salty taste, and somewhat acid. The amount passed in 24 hours averages between a quart and a quart and a half. Normally within the urine are found specific amounts of urea, chloride salts, sulfates and phosphates, hormones, pigments, sulphur, and a number of other products thrown off by the body. The most important constituents that indicate abnormality are blood, pus, sugar, albumin, fat, chyle, bacteria, and other cells. —*incontinence of u.* The inability to hold urine in the bladder. —*residual u.* Any unusual amount of urine that remains in the bladder after urination. In the female this is commonly caused by a downward bulging of the bladder, often the result of childbirth or pressure from tumors of the womb. In the male, enlargement of the prostate and bladder disease are the commonest causes. —*retention of u.* The inability to pass urine. —*suppression of u.* When the kidneys suddenly stop excreting urine.

urogenital (*you-roh-jehn'ih-tuhl*). Relating to the urinary and genital organs.

urologist. A specialist in the diseases and treatment of the urinary and genital tract in the male and the urinary tract in the female.

urology. The branch of medicine that involves the study and treatment of diseases and defects of the urinary and genital organs in the male and urinary organs in the female.

urticaria (*uhr-tih-kaa'rih-uh*). Hives. A condition of the skin with elevations or welts that are white in the center surrounded by an area of redness. These itch intensely and may appear singly, in crops all over the body, or in one area alone. May last from a very short time to days, weeks, or months. —*allergic u.* Due to allergy, most frequently from eating things to which the individual is allergic. Welts also occur as a result of inhalation; contact with, or injection of things to which the individual is allergic; or allergy to germs that are present in the individual's body in teeth, tonsils, and sinuses; or physical agents, as heat, light, cold, mechanical irritation; or to emotional disturbance.

uterine (*you'tuhr-ihn*). Relating to the womb.

uterography (*you-tuhr-ahg'ruh-fih*). X-ray of the womb cavity after the injection of an oil (usually containing iodine) that is opaque to X-rays and results in an outline of the womb cavity and its walls on the X-ray film.

uterus (*you'tuhr-uhss*). The womb. A pear-shaped organ consisting mostly of muscle. Normally three inches long, two wide, and one thick. It is divided into the *fundus*, an upper broad portion; the *body* or *corpus*, that gradually narrows down to the *neck*, commonly called the *cervix*, and extends partially into the upper section of the vagina. The opening of the womb is in communication with the vagina. The inner part of the womb is lined with mucous membrane. The entire organ is suspended in the lower abdomen, the pelvis, by means of three sets of ligaments. The Fallopian tubes enter the womb, one on each side of the fundus. The womb's chief function is to receive and hold the fertilized egg cell during development of the infant and to expel the mature infant during labor. —*gravid u.* A pregnant womb. —*infantile u.* A normally formed but undeveloped womb. —*retroversion of u.* A malposition of the womb in which it is bent backward.

uvula (*you'vyuh-luh*). A small, cone-shaped tongue of tissue that hangs down from the soft palate in the back of the mouth.

V

vaccination. 1. Specifically, the procedure for protection against smallpox by working into the skin the virus that causes cowpox. 2. Injection with any germ to produce immunity against the disease it causes.

vaccine (*vaak'seen*). A suspension of germs used as an injection for prevention of a specific disease. Ordinarily, the germs are either killed or made weaker through chemicals, heat, or vibration before use as a vaccine. They are then suspended in a liquid and counted under the microscope so that definite strengths of the vaccine can be determined. Vaccine is often confused with extracts that are usually simple water solutions of materials, as those used in hay fever injections; with toxin-antitoxins and toxoids that are altered poisons of the bacteria rather than the bacteria themselves and are used against tetanus and diphtheria. —*autogenous v.* A vaccine made from germs obtained from the patient himself, as from the sinuses, teeth, throat, nose, bowel. —*BCG* (*Bacillus Calmette-Guerin*). A vaccine made from weakened tuberculosis germs obtained from humans. Used to develop immunity against tuberculosis. —*brucella v.* One used in the treatment of undulant fever. —*pertussis v.* One made from the germ of whooping cough, *Hemophilus pertussis*, for the treatment and prevention of whooping cough. —*rabies v.* A vaccine made from the spinal cords of animals suffering from rabies and that therefore have the virus within them. Used exclusively as a preventative of rabies after the bite of a rabid animal. —*smallpox v.* A suspension of the virus that produces cowpox in cows obtained from the blisters on the hides of cows infected intentionally with this virus. Smallpox vaccine is used only for the prevention and not for the treatment of smallpox. —*typhoid v.* A suspension of killed typhoid germs used to produce immunity against typhoid fever.

vagina (*vuh-jigh'nuh*). 1. A sheath. 2. The canal that runs from the external female genital organ to surround the neck of the womb. During intercourse, it ensheathes the penis. Its wall consists of muscle, fibrous tissue, and mucous membrane.

vaginismus (*vaaj-ih-nihz'muhss*). Painful spasm of the vagina. —*mental v.* Due to extreme dislike of the sex act.

vaginitis. 1. Inflammation of the vagina. 2. Inflammation of a sheath, as a sheath that surrounds a tendon. —*atrophic v.* After the change of life, natural or induced by surgery, inflammation of the vagina may occur (called *atrophic v.* because the vagina tends to shrink). —*senile v.* Another name for *atrophic v.* —*trichomonas vaginalis v.* Inflammation of the vagina caused by *trichomonas vaginalis* that is found in the secretions and canal of the vagina in this condition.

vagus (*vay'guhss*). The tenth and largest cranial nerve that has its origin in the brain and carries impulses to many organs in the head, neck, chest, and abdomen.

valgus. A term that indicates position. When used of the foot it means a turning outward. When used of the knee it may mean either knock-kneed or bowlegged. If of the hip it means an increase in the angle between the hip and the thighbone. When used of the great toe it indicates a turning of that toe toward the others. Ordinarily when used alone it refers to the foot.

valve. A structure in a passageway that prevents the backward flowing of its contents. Valves are present in the heart, veins, arteries, at strategic points in the intestinal tract, the bladder, and other areas.

valvotomy (*vaal-vaht'uh-mih*). The surgical cutting into a valve, especially in the rectum.

valvulitis (*vaal-vyuh-ligh'tihss*). Inflammation of a valve, particularly a heart valve.

valvulotomy. The surgical incision of a heart valve.

varicella. Chicken pox.

varicocele (*vaar'ih-koh-seel*). A widening of the veins that surround the testes in the male, or the ovaries in the female. This widening eventually forms a swelling that is soft and elastic and feels like a collection of worms.

varicose. A word used to describe vessels that are knotted, swollen, and tortuous, as *varicose veins*.

varicotomy. The surgical removal of a varicose vein.

variola (*vuh-righ'uh-luh*). Smallpox.

variolation (*vaar-ih-uh-lay'shuhn*). An old method of prevention of smallpox consisting of inoculating or snuffing the smallpox scabs. This is a dangerous practice and is forbidden in most parts of the world.

varus. A term that indicates position. When used of the foot it means a turning in; of the knee, bowlegged; of the hip, a decreased angle between the thigh bone and the hip; of the great toe, a turning of that toe from the other toes. When used alone it ordinarily refers to the foot.

vas, *pl.* vasa. 1. A vessel. 2. Passageway.

vascular. Relating to, made of, or supplied with vessels. Most often refers to blood vessels.

vasectomy. The surgical removal of part or all of the tube that conducts the semen from the testes to the penis. Often used for sterilization in the male.

vasoconstrictor. Causing a narrowing of diameter of blood vessels; any agent or nerve that does so.

vasodepressor. Any agent or nerve that relaxes the blood vessels, thereby increasing their diameter and lowering blood pressure.

vasodilator. Any agent that produces a widening of the diameter of blood vessels.

vasomotor (*vay-soh-moh'tuhr*). Regulating the narrowing (*vasoconstriction*) and widening (*vasodilation*) of the blood vessels.

vasotomy (*vaa-saht'uh-mih*). A surgical cutting into the tube that conducts semen from the testis to the penis.

vein. A blood vessel that carries blood to the heart. In contradistinction to an artery that carries blood from the heart out to the body.

venereal. Relating to, or caused by, sexual intercourse.

venesection (*vehn-uh-sehk'shuhn*). Bleeding; the removal of blood from the body by cutting a vein, ordinarily done by a needle and syringe.

venipuncture. The puncture of a vein surgically, as the introduction of a needle.

ventricle (*vehn'trih-kuhl*). A small cavity or pouch. —*left v. of the heart.* That which forces the blood through the large artery, the aorta, thence throughout the body. —*right v. of the heart.* That which forces blood into the lungs through the pulmonary artery.

ventriculogram (*vehn-trihk'yuh-luh-graam*). An X-ray of the brain that is made after introduction of air or a material

opaque to X-ray into the cavities of the brain through trephine openings in the skull. The purpose is to outline the
brain cavities (*cerebral ventricles*) and determine the presence of disease.

vernal. Relating to spring, as *vernal catarrh*, an inflammation
of the eyes that is seasonal.

verruca (*veh-roo'kuh*). Wart. —*v. plana juvenilis*. A small,
flat, smooth wart, most often seen in children on the back
of the hands and the face. —*v. plantaris*. A wart of the sole
of the foot. Because of pressure in this region, it grows inward and is quite painful. It is often covered with a callus.
—*v. senilis*. A brownish wart seen on the face, chest, and back
of older people, usually greasy and scaly, and may at times
become cancerous. —*v. vulgaris*. The ordinary wart that is
caused by a virus, more common in children, ordinarily about
the fingernails, arms, and legs.

version. Turning; the turning of the infant within the womb
by the obstetrician during delivery to a more favorable position.

vertebra. One of 33 bones that make up the spinal or ver-
tebral column, commonly known as the spine. These are
divided into seven *cervical* in the neck; twelve *thoracic* or
dorsal in the back of the chest to which ribs are attached;
five *lumbar* in the low back, extending between the lower
border of the chest cage and the top of the hip bone; five
sacral that are joined together and are called the *sacrum*, uniting the hip bones behind; and four *coccygeal*, united together
as the *coccyx*, or the tail bone.

vertex. The crown of the head.

vertical. Relating to the vertex.

vertigo. Dizziness. A sense of lack of balance due to a number of conditions, as diseases of the ear, eyes, brain, stomach,
blood. —*labyrinthine v*. A term synonymous with *Meniere's
syndrome*. Consists of dizziness, pallor, ringing in the ears,
rapid movements of the eyes, nausea, vomiting. Due to in-

flammation of that part of the internal ear that has to do with balance.

vesica. A bladder, as the urinary bladder, *v. urinaria.*

vesicant (*vehs'ih-kuhnt*). Blistering or a blistering agent. Also refers to a gas used in warfare that causes blistering, as *mustard gas* and *lewisite.*

vesicle. 1. A small bladder; especially a tiny pouch containing fluid. 2. A small blister of the skin as a cold blister or a chicken pox blister.

vessel. A tube or passageway for conveying lymph or blood, such as blood vessel, lymph vessel.

vestibule. A foyer; antechamber; or approach, as *v. of the mouth* is the space bounded by the gums and teeth inside, the lips and cheeks outside.

villus. A microscopic projection from a surface, especially an internal surface. —*intestinal v.* Minute projections from the lining mucous membrane of the small intestine that are involved in the absorption of emulsified fats. —*synovial v.* Projections from the lining membrane of a joint cavity into the cavity itself.

virilism. 1. Maleness. The development of male characteristics in the female. 2. A form of *pseudohermaphroditism* in which the individual is a female but has external genitals that look in varying degrees like those of a male.

virology. The specialty that deals with viruses and the diseases they produce.

virulence. Poisonousness; the power of injuring; infectiousness; endangering life; the power of a germ to produce disease.

virus. Generally means any poison, particularly of an infectious disease. Specifically refers to a group of disease-producing agents smaller than the ordinary germ, any of which, known as *ultraviruses*, are not visible under the light microscope. The virus may be a living form. There are many diseases caused by viruses in man, as rabies, infantile paralysis, various forms of encephalitis, the common cold, smallpox, chicken pox, measles, mumps, influenza, shingles, yellow fever, and others.

viscus (*vihss'kuhss*), *pl. viscera.* Any of the organs within the four great body cavities, the cranium (skull cavity), thorax (the chest cavity), abdomen (belly cavity), or pelvis (the cavity enclosed by the hip bones). Especially refers to an organ within the abdominal cavity.

vitamin. One of a group of substances, organic in nature, present in minute and variable amounts in natural food, necessary for the normal growth and the continuation of life in animals and man. They are usually effective in small amounts and unlike food do not furnish energy themselves but are essential in deriving energy from food and in regulating the processes of energy-exchange in the individual. The known vitamins are vitamin A; the vitamin-B complex, consisting of six separate vitamins; vitamins C, D, E, H, K, and P. Each has a specific function that is vital for normal growth and life.

vitiligo (*viht-ih-ligh'goh*). A skin disease in which there are various sized and shaped areas lacking the normal color, with borders of deeper than normal color. These areas are more noticeable in parts that are exposed to the air. Also called *leukoderma, piebald skin.*

vitreous. Refers to the gelatine-like, transparent material that fills the larger part of the eyeball behind the lens.

voice. The sounds that are produced by the vibration of the vocal cords and modified by various resonating organs, such as the voice box itself, the nose, the mouth.

vomer. A thin sheet of bone that forms the upper part of the partition dividing the nose into two chambers.

vomitus. Vomited matter.

vulva. The female genital.

vulvectomy. The surgical removal of the female genital organ.

vulvitis. Inflammation of the female genital.

vulvovaginitis (*vul-vuh-vaaj-ih-nigh'tihss*). Inflammation of the female genital organ and the vagina at the same time.

W

wart. A horny, overgrown projection of the skin.

weeping. 1. The flowing of tears. 2. The leakage of a fluid. 3. The seeping of a fluid from a raw surface.

wen. A cyst of the oil glands of the skin; so-called commonly when it occurs on the scalp. Also called *sebaceous cyst*.

wheal. An affection of the skin characterized by swelling sharply marked off from the rest of the skin. It varies from pinhead size to cantaloupe or larger. The swelling comes and goes and is accompanied by itching, burning, or tingling. Characteristic of hives, but may occur after insect or animal bites.

wheeze. A sighing or whistling sound heard during breathing. At times is audible at some distance from the patient and other times only through the stethoscope. Means obstruction of one or more of the air passages, often heard in asthma.

whitlow. An obsolete term for any pus-forming infection on the end of a finger or toe.

whooping cough. An infectious disease most frequently occurring in children due to an inflammation of air passages, and characterized by attacks of severe coughing that end in a loud whooping intake of breath. Also called *pertussis*.

womb. *See* UTERUS.

wound. The interruption of the normal continuity of a body surface.

wrist. The part that links the forearm and the hand.

wryneck. Another term for *torticollis*.

X

xanthelasma (*zaan-theh-laaz'muh*). A yellowish or orange-colored, flat or elevated patch of skin, pinhead to bean size, occurring on the eyelid. A type of *xanthoma*.

xanthoma (*zaan-thoh'muh*). A flat or slightly elevated new growth of skin, pinhead to bean size, yellowish or orange in color, caused by disturbance in the ability of the body to break down fats. —*x. diabeticorum*. Dull red, solid, slightly raised patches of skin; most often in the palms and soles. Seen sometimes though rarely in diabetes. —*x. tuberosum*. The commonest type of *xanthoma* characterized by groups of elevations on the skin, yellow in color, that may also occur in internal organs, about tendons and thus give rise to a great variety of symptoms.

xanthosis. A yellowish discoloration of the skin due to the deposition of a pigment known as *carotene*, the result of eating large quantities of sweet potatoes, squash, carrots, and other similar vegetables. During the war this condition was seen following the use of atabrine in the treatment and prevention of malaria. Shortly after cessation of the drug or eating the implicated foods the skin clears up.

xeroderma (*zih-roh-duhr'muh*). 1. Unusual dryness of the skin. 2. A specific disease in which the skin is dry, tough, discolored, and comes off in a fine, branny scale. Also called *ichthyosis*. —*x. pigmentosum*. An unusual disease with a family tendency that begins in childhood and is characterized by spots of pigment spread over the skin, dryness and tightness of the skin, and spider-webbing of the small blood vessels. These changes are most common in the skin areas exposed to sunlight. In a short time, wartlike elevations appear in the skin that may eventually develop into cancer and the skin takes on many of the characteristics of the skin of the aged. This condition has many names, the commonest being *Kaposi's disease.*

xerophthalmia (*zih-rahf-thaal'mih-uh*). A condition in which the lining membrane of the lid and the eyeball is dry and thickened. May follow on chronic conjunctivitis; disease of the tear-producing and conveying apparatus; or a deficiency in vitamin A.

xerosis. A condition of dryness, especially of the skin, or of the lining tissue of the lids and eyeballs.

xiphoid (*zihf'oyd*). Sword-shaped. Refers to the lower end of the breastbone.

Y

yaws. An infectious disease of the tropics caused by a germ, *Treponema pertenue*, that belongs to the syphilis family. This disease, unlike syphilis, is not venereal. The germ enters the body through the skin and is thought to be introduced by certain flies. The disease itself, at first, involves the skin with an initial "mother yaw" and is followed by crops of raspberry-like elevations over the entire body. Late in the disease, skin and bones may be destroyed. If in this stage the nose and the mouth are involved, the condition is called *gangosa.*

yellow fever. An infectious disease of sudden onset particularly prevalent in the American tropics and subtropics. It is caused by a virus carried to man by a mosquito, *Aedes aegypti.* Several hours to days after being bitten, the individual develops a fever up to 105°, chills, pains in the head, back and limbs, vomiting, and scanty urine. A short period of relief may follow, then the fever recurs, jaundice discolors skin and eyes yellow, black vomit due to the presence of blood becomes profuse, bleeding from the intestines may appear. Death often results.

Z

zonesthesia. A sensation as of a tight girdle about the waist. Also called *girdle pain.*

zooerastea (*zoh-oh-ehr-aass'tih-uh*). Sexual intercourse with an animal.

zoopsia (*zoh-ahp'sih-uh*). Hallucinations, illusions, dreams that are peopled with animals. Occurs often in delirium tremens.

zoster. A disease of sudden onset with pain or burning and groups of small blisters in the course of a nerve. Also called *shingles, herpes zoster.*

zygoma. The cheek bone.

THE VITAMINS

(common and less common names, and dietary sources)

names	chief dietary sources

VITAMIN A

anti-xerophthalmia factor
axerophthal
antixerotic factor
vitamin A_1

Apricots, asparagus, beet greens, broccoli, butter, carrots, cantaloupe, chard, cheese, collards, dandelion greens, eggs, kale, liver, margarine, mustard greens, spinach, squash, sweet potatoes, turnip greens, tomatoes.

VITAMIN B_c

pteroylglutamic acid
folic acid
antianemia factor
vitamin M
folacin
factor U,L
casei factor
norite eluate factor

Asparagus, bananas, dried lima beans, green beans, wax beans, beef liver, beef, beets, beet greens, whole wheat bread, broccoli, cantaloupe, carrots, cauliflower, cheese, chicken, eggs, endive, ham, kale, lettuce, mushrooms, oranges, oysters, parsley, peanuts, green peas, pork, white potatoes, radishes, salmon, spinach, Swiss chard, tomatoes, veal, watermelon, whole wheat, wheat germ.

VITAMIN B_x

para-aminobenzoic acid
chromotrichia factor
anti-gray hair factor
vitamin H'

Yeast, liver, wheat germ.

VITAMIN B_1

thiamine
aneurin

Bacon, kidney and lima beans, bologna, whole wheat or enriched white bread,

anti-neuritic factor
anti-beriberi factor

whole grain cornmeal, enriched farina, buckwheat flour, whole grain rye, soy or enriched white flour, heart, whole or skimmed milk, oatmeal, peanuts, green or split peas, pecans, pork, brown rice, soy beans, walnuts, wheat germ.

VITAMIN B₂

riboflavin
vitamin G
lactoflavin
ovoflavin
hepatoflavin
verdoflavin

Almonds, avocadoes, dry beans, dried beef, bologna, enriched white or whole wheat bread, cheddar cheese, whole grain cornmeal, eggs, enriched farina, soy flour, heart, kale, lamb, fresh liver, liver sausage, dry or evaporated milk, salmon, turnip greens, wheat germ.

VITAMIN B₆

pyridoxine
pyridoxal
pyridoxamine
pyridoximers
eluate factor
anti-acrodynia factor
adermin
factor 1,Y
anti-dermatitis factor

Apples, bananas, dried lima beans, beef liver, beef heart, beef, whole wheat bread, cabbage, cantaloupe, cauliflower, cheese, chicken, eggs, halibut, lettuce, whole milk, molasses, oranges, fresh or dried peas, peanuts, pork, white potatoes, sweet potatoes, spinach, turnips, veal, wheat germ.

VITAMIN B₁₂

anti-pernicious anemia factor

Milk, cheese, meats, egg yolk.

VITAMIN C

ascorbic acid
anti-scorbutic factor
cevitamic acid

Asparagus, green lima beans, broccoli, Brussels sprouts, cabbage, cantaloupe, cauliflower, chard, collards, dandelion greens, grapefruit, kale, lemon, lime, fresh liver, mustard greens, okra, orange, green peas, green pepper, pineapple, radish, rutabaga, spinach, strawberries, sweet potatoes, tangerines, tomatoes, turnip greens and turnip.

VITAMIN D

antirachitic vitamin
calciferol
activated 7-dehydrocholesterol

Butter, cod liver oil, eggs, halibut liver oil, herring, calf or pork liver, mackerel, evaporated or fortified milk, canned salmon or tuna.

VITAMIN E

anti-sterility factor
fertility vitamin
tocopherol

Beef liver, dry beans, butter, coconut oil, cornmeal, corn oil, cottonseed oil, eggs, margarine, oatmeal, peanut oil, green peas, sweet potatoes, brown rice, soy bean oil, turnip greens.

VITAMIN H

anti-egg-white injury factor
biotin
coenzyme R
bios IIb
skin factor
factors S; W; X

Bananas, dried lima beans, beef, carrots, cauliflower, cheese, chicken, chocolate, corn, egg, grapefruit, halibut, beef liver, milk, molasses, mushroom, onions, oysters, peas, peanuts, pork, salmon, spinach, strawberries, tomatoes, whole wheat.

VITAMIN K

anti-hemorrhagic factor
Koagulationsvitamin
phylloquinone
vitamin K_1

Cabbage, carrots, cauliflower, cereals, pork liver, green peas, spinach, green and ripe tomatoes.

VITAMIN P

citrin
permeability vitamin

Lemon and lemon peel, orange, grape, plum, black currants.

CHOLINE

bilineurine
fagine
amanitine
sinkaline

Asparagus, snap and soy beans, beef, bologna, cabbage, carrots, cheddar cheese, germ corn, egg yolk, lamb and lamb kidney, beef and pork liver, liver sausage, milk, rolled oats, peanuts, peas, pecans, pork, white potatoes, spinach, trout, turnips, wheat germ.

INOSITOL

mouse anti-alopecia factor
bios I
muscle sugar

Bacon, dried lima beans, beef brain and heart and liver, white and whole wheat bread, cantaloupe, cauliflower, chocolate, grapefruit, ham, lamb, lettuce, mutton, onion, oranges, peach, peanut, dried and green peas, sweet potatoes, raisin, strawberry, watermelon, wheat germ and whole wheat.

NICOTINIC ACID

niacin
nicotinamide
pellagra-preventive factor
  (P.P. factor)
antipellagra factor
anti-black tongue factor

Almonds, avocadoes, beef, bologna, enriched white and whole wheat bread, chicken, yellow cornmeal, fish, enriched wheat flour, whole wheat flour, fresh heart, lamb, fresh liver, liver sausage, peanut, green and split peas, pork, brown and converted rice, canned sardines, tomato, fresh tongue, canned tuna, turkey, veal, wheat cereals, wheat germ.

PANTOTHENIC ACID

pantothen
filtrate factor
chick anti-dermatitis factor
chick anti-pellagra factor
factor II
anti chromotrichia (gray hair)
  factor

Dried lima beans, beef liver, brain, heart and muscle, whole wheat and white bread, broccoli, cauliflower, cheese, chicken, egg, lamb, whole milk, mushroom, oats, orange, oyster, fresh and dried peas, peanuts, pork, white and sweet potatoes, salmon, soy bean, veal, whole wheat and wheat germ.

UNSATURATED FATTY ACIDS (ESSENTIAL)

vitamin F (?)

Butter, cod liver oil, corn germ oil, cottonseed oil, lard, linseed oil, olive oil, palm oil, peanut oil, soy bean oil.

Several other vitamins are known, but their importance in body functioning is only now being determined. Among these are: Adenylic acid and streptogenin.

SOME IMPORTANT HORMONES

source	hormone	important natural function
ADRENAL GLAND Cortex	Adrenosterone	Stimulates masculine characteristics.
	Estrone	Stimulates the lining tissue of the womb to undergo all of the typical changes occurring during the menstrual cycle.
	Progesterone	Influences the lining tissue of the womb toward those changes necessary for pregnancy.
	Corticosterones (there are six of these)	These are necessary for the maintenance of life; have to do with salt balance and the breakdown of starches; operate in contending with stress and various other deleterious body situations; influence the efficiency of muscles.
Medulla	Epinephrine (or adrenalin)	Stimulates the action of the sympathetic nervous system, readying the body for fight or flight.
INTESTINE (MUCOSA)	Cholecystokinin	Stimulates the gall bladder to contract.

	Enterocrinin	Stimulates the glands in the mucosa of the small intestine to contract.
	Enterogastrone	Prevents contraction and secretion of the stomach.
	Secretin	Stimulates the production and flow of juice from the pancreas.
OVARY	Estrone	See under Adrenal cortex.
	Estradiol	Action similar to estrone.
	Progesterone	See under Adrenal cortex.
PANCREAS	Insulin	Regulates the breakdown of starches in tissues and the storage of sugar in the liver as glycogen.
PARA-THYROID	Parathyroid hormone (or parathormone, or parathyrin)	Controls the utilization and disposal of calcium and phosphorus.
PITUITARY Anterior lobe	Luteinizing hormone (LH)	Stimulates the formation of luteal bodies in the ovary, the persistence of which is necessary for pregnancy to proceed normally.
	Follicle stimulating hormone (FSH)	In the female: increases size of the ovary and also the growth of follicles within the ovary. These follicles are the sites in which the ova grow and from which the ova are expelled (by rupture of the follicle) into the abdominal cavity and thence into the "tubes." In the male: Increases size of the testes and stimulates the formation and maturation of sperm.

	Prolactin	Stimulates breast milk production.
	Growth hormone	Influence bodily growth.
	Thyrotrophic hormone	Regulates the secretion of the thyroid gland.
	Adrenotrophic hormone ACTH	Regulates the secretions of the adrenal cortex.
Posterior lobe	Posterior pituitary hormones (pitocin, pitressin and others)	Helps to regulate blood pressure; stimulates the contraction of the womb; tends to prevent the passage of water through the kidneys.
PLACENTA	Estrone	See under Adrenal cortex.
	Estriol	Action similar to estrone.
	Estradiol	Action similar to estrone.
	Progesterone	See under Adrenal gland.
	Pregnant mare's serum hormone (PMS)	Causes effects of both LH & FSH.
TESTES	Testosterone	Stimulates masculine characteristics.
THYROID	Thyroxin	Controls the metabolic rate.

FOR WOMEN

HEIGHT (with shoes on) Feet Inches	WEIGHT IN POUNDS ACCORDING TO FRAME (as Ordinarily Dressed)		
	SMALL FRAME	MEDIUM FRAME	LARGE FRAME
4 11	104–111	110–118	117–127
5 0	105–113	112–120	119–129
5 1	107–115	114–122	121–131
5 2	110–118	117–125	124–135
5 3	113–121	120–128	127–138
5 4	116–125	124–132	131–142
5 5	119–128	127–135	133–145
5 6	123–132	130–140	138–150
5 7	126–136	134–144	142–154
5 8	129–139	137–147	145–158
5 9	133–143	141–151	149–162
5 10	136–147	145–155	152–166
5 11	139–150	148–158	155–169

FOR MEN

HEIGHT (with shoes on) Feet Inches	WEIGHT IN POUNDS ACCORDING TO FRAME (as Ordinarily Dressed)		
	SMALL FRAME	MEDIUM FRAME	LARGE FRAME
5 2	116–125	124–133	131–142
5 3	119–128	127–136	133–144
5 4	122–132	130–140	137–149
5 5	126–136	134–144	141–153
5 6	129–139	137–147	145–157
5 7	133–143	141–151	149–162
5 8	136–147	145–156	153–166
5 9	140–151	149–160	157–170
5 10	144–155	153–164	161–175
5 11	148–159	157–168	165–180
6 0	152–164	161–173	169–185
6 1	157–169	166–178	174–190
6 2	163–175	171–184	179–196
6 3	168–180	176–189	184–202

OBSTETRIC TABLE

January....	1 2 3 4 5 6 7 8 9 10 11 12 13 14 15 16 17 18 19 20 21 22 23 24 25 26 27 28 29 30 31	
October.....	8 9 10 11 12 13 14 15 16 17 18 19 20 21 22 23 24 25 26 27 28 29 30 31 1 2 3 4 5 6 7	November
February....	1 2 3 4 5 6 7 8 9 10 11 12 13 14 15 16 17 18 19 20 21 22 23 24 25 26 27 28 29	
November...	8 9 10 11 12 13 14 15 16 17 18 19 20 21 22 23 24 25 26 27 28 29 30 1 2 3 4 5	December
March.......	1 2 3 4 5 6 7 8 9 10 11 12 13 14 15 16 17 18 19 20 21 22 23 24 25 26 27 28 29 30 31	
December..	6 7 8 9 10 11 12 13 14 15 16 17 18 19 20 21 22 23 24 25 26 27 28 29 30 31 1 2 3 4 5	January
April.......	1 2 3 4 5 6 7 8 9 10 11 12 13 14 15 16 17 18 19 20 21 22 23 24 25 26 27 28 29 30	
January.....	6 7 8 9 10 11 12 13 14 15 16 17 18 19 20 21 22 23 24 25 26 27 28 29 30 31 1 2 3 4	February
May.........	1 2 3 4 5 6 7 8 9 10 11 12 13 14 15 16 17 18 19 20 21 22 23 24 25 26 27 28 29 30 31	
February...	5 6 7 8 9 10 11 12 13 14 15 16 17 18 f9 20 21 22 23 24 25 26 27 28 1 2 3 4 5 6 7	March
June.........	1 2 3 4 5 6 7 8 9 10 11 12 13 14 15 16 17 18 19 20 21 22 23 24 25 26 27 28 29 30	
March......	8 9 10 11 12 13 14 15 16 17 18 19 20 21 22 23 24 25 26 27 28 29 30 31 1 2 3 4 5 6	April
July.........	1 2 3 4 5 6 7 8 9 10 11 12 13 14 15 16 17 18 19 20 21 22 23 24 25 26 27 28 29 30 31	
April......	7 8 9 10 11 12 13 14 15 16 17 18 19 20 21 22 23 24 25 26 27 28 29 30 1 2 3 4 5 6 7	May
August......	1 2 3 4 5 6 7 8 9 10 11 12 13 14 15 16 17 18 19 20 21 22 23 24 25 26 27 28 29 30 31	
May........	8 9 10 11 12 13 14 15 16 17 18 19 20 21 22 23 24 25 26 27 28 29 30 31 1 2 3 4 5 6 7	June
September..	1 2 3 4 5 6 7 8 9 10 11 12 13 14 15 16 17 18 19 20 21 22 23 24 25 26 27 28 29 30	
June........	8 9 10 11 12 13 14 15 16 17 18 19 20 21 22 23 24 25 26 27 28 29 30 1 2 3 4 5 6 7	July
October....	1 2 3 4 5 6 7 8 9 10 11 12 13 14 15 16 17 18 19 20 21 22 23 24 25 26 27 28 29 30 31	
July........	8 9 10 11 12 13 14 15 16 17 18 19 20 21 22 23 24 25 26 27 28 29 30 31 1 2 3 4 5 6 7	August
November..	1 2 3 4 5 6 7 8 9 10 11 12 13 14 15 16 17 18 19 20 21 22 23 24 25 26 27 28 29 30	
August.....	8 9 10 11 12 13 14 15 16 17 18 19 20 21 22 23 24 25 26 27 28 29 30 31 1 2 3 4 5 6	September
December..	1 2 3 4 5 6 7 8 9 10 11 12 13 14 15 16 17 18 19 20 21 22 23 24 25 26 27 28 29 30 31	
September..	7 8 9 10 11 12 13 14 15 16 17 18 19 20 21 22 23 24 25 26 27 28 29 30 1 2 3 4 5 6 7	October

The numbers in the first line represent the first day of the last menstrual period; those directly below the probable date of parturition.

THE HIPPOCRATIC OATH

Estimated to have been written between the fifth and first centuries B. C., and still administered in some medical schools, this oath represents the spirit of medicine.

I swear by Apollo Physician, by Asclepius, by Health, by Panacea, and by all gods and goddesses, making them my witnesses, that I will carry out, according to my ability and judgment this oath and indenture: To hold my teacher in this art equal to my own parents; to make him partner in my livelihood; when he is in need of money to share mine with him; to consider his family as my own brothers, and to teach them this art, if they want to learn it, without fee or indenture; to impart precept, oral instruction, and all other instruction to my own sons, to the sons of my teacher, and to indentured pupils who have taken the physician's oath, but to nobody else. I will use treatment to help the sick according to my ability and judgment, but never with a view to injury and wrongdoing. Neither will I administer a poison to anybody when asked to do so, nor will I suggest such a course. Similarly I will not give a woman a pessary to cause abortion. But I will keep pure and holy both my life and my art. I will not use the knife, not even, verily, on sufferers from the stone, but I will give place to such as are craftsmen therein. Into whatsoever house I enter, I will enter to help the sick, and I will abstain from all intentional wrongdoing and harm, especially from abusing the bodies of man or woman, bond or free. And whatsoever I shall see or hear in the course of my profession, as well as outside my profession in my intercourse with men, if it be what should not be published abroad, I will never divulge, holding such things to be holy secrets. Now if I carry out this oath and break it not, may I gain forever reputation among all men for my life and my art; but if I transgress it and forswear myself, may the opposite befall me.

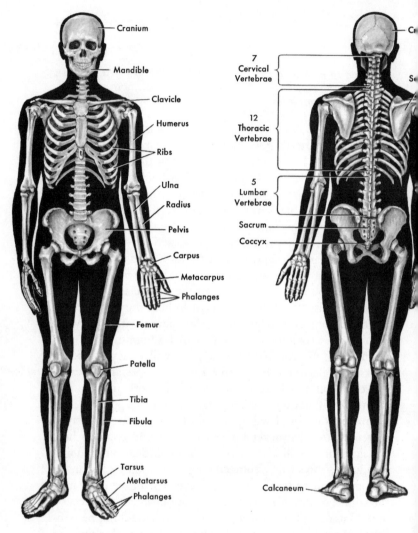

FRONT VIEW

BACK VIEW

THE HUMAN SKELETON

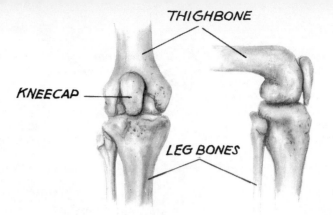

KNEE JOINT

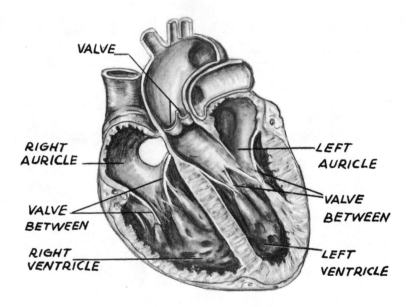

THE CHAMBERS AND VALVES OF THE HEART

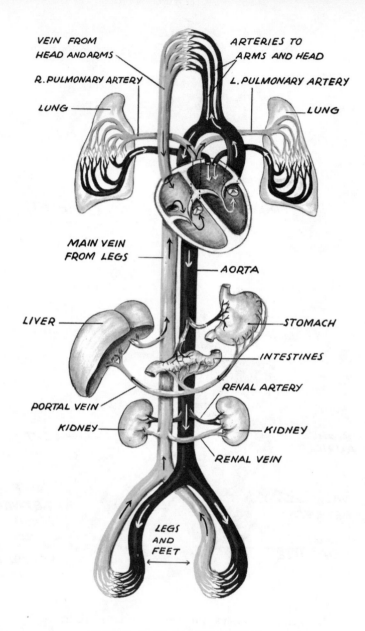

VEIN FROM HEAD AND ARMS

ARTERIES TO ARMS AND HEAD

R. PULMONARY ARTERY

L. PULMONARY ARTERY

LUNG

LUNG

MAIN VEIN FROM LEGS

AORTA

LIVER

STOMACH

INTESTINES

RENAL ARTERY

PORTAL VEIN

KIDNEY

KIDNEY

RENAL VEIN

LEGS AND FEET

GENERAL PLAN OF CIRCULATION

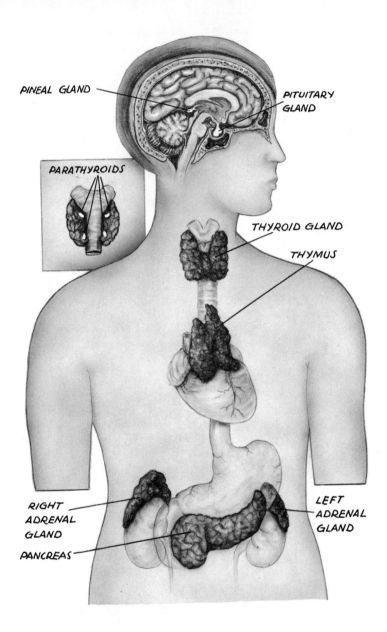

PINEAL GLAND

PITUITARY GLAND

PARATHYROIDS

THYROID GLAND

THYMUS

RIGHT ADRENAL GLAND

LEFT ADRENAL GLAND

PANCREAS

THE ENDOCRINE GLANDS

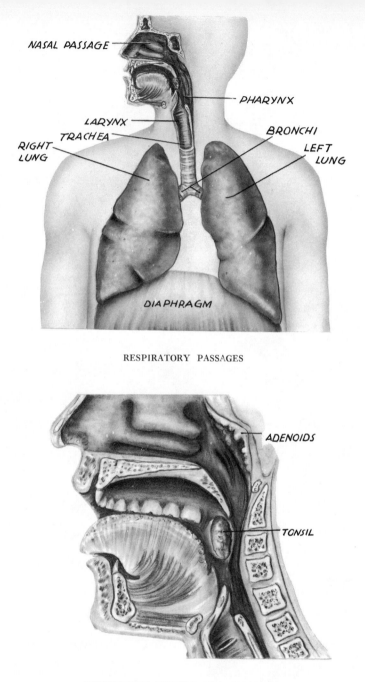

RESPIRATORY PASSAGES

WHERE THE TONSILS ARE LOCATED

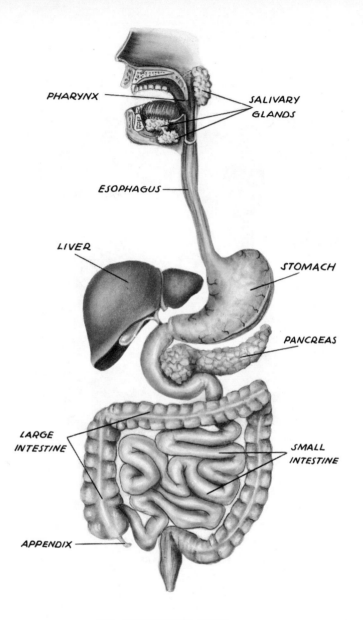

PHARYNX

SALIVARY
GLANDS

ESOPHAGUS

LIVER

STOMACH

PANCREAS

LARGE
INTESTINE

SMALL
INTESTINE

APPENDIX

THE ALIMENTARY CANAL

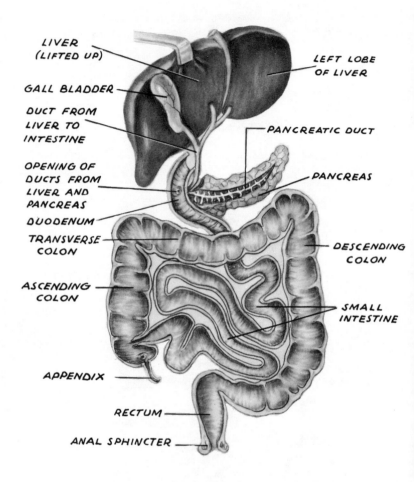

LIVER
(LIFTED UP)

GALL BLADDER

DUCT FROM
LIVER TO
INTESTINE

OPENING OF
DUCTS FROM
LIVER AND
PANCREAS

DUODENUM

TRANSVERSE
COLON

ASCENDING
COLON

APPENDIX

RECTUM

ANAL SPHINCTER

LEFT LOBE
OF LIVER

PANCREATIC DUCT

PANCREAS

DESCENDING
COLON

SMALL
INTESTINE

THE INTESTINES

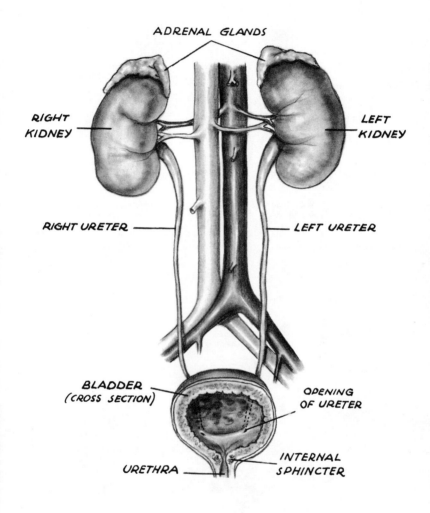

ADRENAL GLANDS

RIGHT
KIDNEY

LEFT
KIDNEY

RIGHT URETER

LEFT URETER

BLADDER
(CROSS SECTION)

OPENING
OF URETER

URETHRA

INTERNAL
SPHINCTER

THE KIDNEYS

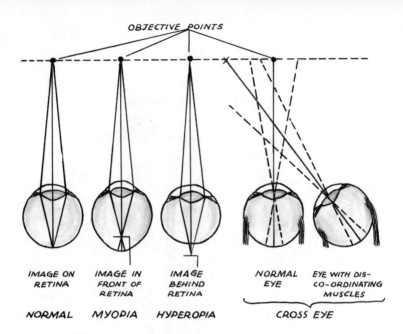

OBJECTIVE POINTS

| IMAGE ON RETINA | IMAGE IN FRONT OF RETINA | IMAGE BEHIND RETINA | NORMAL EYE | EYE WITH DIS-CO-ORDINATING MUSCLES |
| NORMAL | MYOPIA | HYPEROPIA | CROSS EYE | |

DIFFERENCE BETWEEN NORMAL AND FAULTY VISION

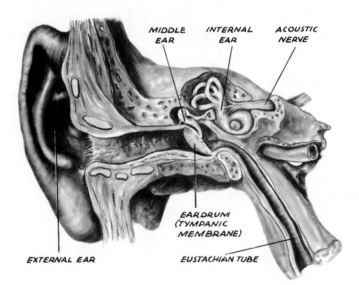

MIDDLE EAR INTERNAL EAR ACOUSTIC NERVE

EARDRUM (TYMPANIC MEMBRANE)

EXTERNAL EAR EUSTACHIAN TUBE

THE EXTERNAL, MIDDLE, AND INTERNAL EAR

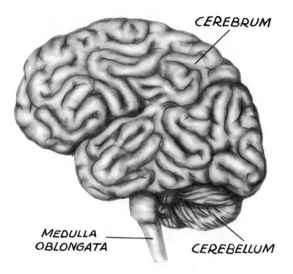

CEREBRUM

MEDULLA
OBLONGATA

CEREBELLUM

THE BRAIN

INDEX AND CROSS-REFERENCE GUIDE

Main entries in SMALL CAPITALS are selected key words. Those interested in any of these topics will find listed with them other main entries offering additional information on the subject. The other index entries refer the reader to those key words under which the particular topic, not itself a main entry, is discussed.

thematosis, parasympathetic, periarteritis nodosa, permeability, photosensitization, poison ivy, poison oak, poison sumac, pollen, pollenosis, pruritis, purpura, pyrethrum flowers, ragweed, rheumatism, rhinitis, rhonchus, rose fever, sick headache, timothy, Trichophyton, tuberculin, urticaria, vasomotor rhinitis, vernal, vertigo (labyrinthine or Meniere's disease), wheal, wheeze

ALOPECIA, *see also* baldness, calvities, folliculitis decalvans, myxedema, pelada

Appendicitis, *see* abdomen, acute

Appendix, *see* appendectomy, cecostomy, cecum

Appetite, *see* altitude sickness, anorexia, biliousness

AUTONOMIC, *see also* acetylcholine, cholinesterase, medulla oblongata, nervous system, parasympathetic, sympathectomy, vagus

AVITAMINOSIS, *see also* ariboflavinosis, beriberi, cheilosis, glossotrichia, keratitis, maize, malnutrition, marasmus, night blindness, pellagra, rachitic, scurvy, tetany, xerophthalmia

Blackhead, *see* acne, comedo

Bleeding, *see* anemia, bleeding time, dementia, electrocoagulation, hemophilia, hemorrhage, hemostat, ligation, menopause, menstruation, metrorrhagia, pachymeningitis, petechia, plague, prothrombin, purpura, scurvy, shock, styptic, tampon, time, tourniquet, typhoid, venesection

Blood, *see* absorption, acetylcholine, albuminuria, anemia, anoxemia, anoxia, aorta, artery, autolysis, autotransfusion, Ayerza's syndrome, bacillemia, bacteremia, ballistocardiograph, bends, biologicals, birthmark, blast injury, bleb, bleeding time, blood count, blood pressure, blood substitute, blood typing, bovine, bronze diabetes, brucellosis, capillary, cholesterol, circulation time, clotting time, congestion, coronary, corpuscle, creatinine, crenation, diastole, extravasation, filaria, flush, gangrene, hemarthrosis, hematemesis, hematic, hematinic, hematocolpos, hematocrit, hematologist, hematology, hematoma, hematuria, hemochromatosis, hemoglobin, hemoglobinemia, hemoglobinometer, hemoglobinuria, hemolysis, hemopericardium, hemophilia, hemoptysis, hemorrhage, hemostat, hemothorax, heparin, hepatomegaly, hormone, hyperemia, hypertension, icterus, immunotransfusion, infarct, infarction, jaundice, lancet, leukemia, liver, malacia, malaria, menorrhagia, menorrhea, menses, metastasis, monocyte, mononucleosis, nephrosclerosis, normocytosis, occult, oscillometer, pancreas, paralysis, penis, permeability, phlebotomy, pile, placenta, plasma, platelet, poison, presystolic, priapism, protein, prothrombin, pulse, purpura, pyruvic acid, rate, ratio, regurgitation, RH factor, rubefacient, sanguine, secrete, secretion, septicemia, serum, shock, sinus, smear, sound, spleen, sputum, stain, stasis, strangulation, suffusion, syncope, syphilis, systole, tension, test, thrombin, thrombinogen, thromboangiitis, thrombocytopenia, thrombophlebitis, thrombus, time, tissue, toxemia, transfusion, trunk, turgor, urine, vein, venesection, ventricle, vertigo, vessel

Boil, *see* abscess, areola, carbuncle, hordeolum, induration, resolution

Bowel(s), *see* diarrhea, dyschizia, evacuant, feces, flux, ileus, lavage, laxative, motion, obstruction, occult, peritonitis, sprue, steatorrhea, stool, test, urgency

Breathing, *see* airway, altitude sickness, bagassosis, cardiac failure, hyperpnea, lung, medulla, menhidrosis, myasthenia, pericarditis, tachypnea, wheeze

Bronchial tubes, *see* aspergillosis, bronchiectasis, bronchitis, bronchogram, bronchopneumonia, bronchoscope, bronchostenosis, emphysema, influenza, inspissate, membrane, movement, mucin, parenchyma

CATALYST, *see also* cholinesterase, enzyme, globulin

CHANCRE, *see also* arsenical, antibiotic, bismuthosis, bubo, specific, spirochete, syphilis, treponema, venereal

Change of life, *see* climacteric, vaginitis

"Charley horse," *see* abasia

CHEMOTHERAPY, *see also* arsenical, aurotherapy, BAL, bromide, calomel, emetine

Childbirth, *see* accouchement, analgesia, breast, convulsion, decidua, labor, pain, pelvis, postpartum

Chills, *see* ague, malaria

Choking, *see* angina, diverticulum, strangulation

CHROMATOSIS, *see also* bronze diabetes, chloasma, chlorosis, denigration, Addison's disease, hemochromatosis, lentigo, melanin, melanosis, sunburn, xanthelasma, xanthoma, xanthosis

CIRRHOSIS, *see also* ascites, alcoholism, cholangitis, bronze diabetes, hemochromatosis, hepatitis, icterus, jaundice, liver

Clot(s), *see* aphasia, coagulant, coagulate, coronary, decidua, fibrin, gangrene, heart block, hemophilia, heparin, liver, necrosis, pain, phlebitic, phlebolith, phlebothrombosis, prothrombin, serum, thromboangiitis, thrombosis, thrombus, time

COITUS, *see also* condom, dyspareunia, ejaculatio, erection, end pleasure, forepleasure, fornication, genitalia, insemination, intromission, orgasm, pareunia, pederasty, penis, phallus, postcoital, priapism, saltpeter, semen, sperm, vagina, vaginismus, venereal, vulva, zooerastea

Color blindness, *see* chromatelopsia

CONVULSION, *see also* alkalosis, chorea, clonus, convulsant, curare, eclampsia, epilepsy, malaria, myotonia, tetanus, tetany

CRETINISM, *see also* endocrinopathy, hypothyroidism, idiocy, obesity, thyroid

DIABETES, *see also* acidosis, carbohydrate, carbuncle, cataract, coma, diuresis, glucose, glycosuria, hemochromatosis, hyperglycemia, ketosis, liver, pancreas, polyphagia, polyuria, retinitis, test, tolerance, urine, xanthoma

DIZZINESS, *see also* air sickness, alcoholism, alkalosis, altitude sickness, anemia, hypoglycemia, inebriation, motion sickness, vertigo

DROPSY, *see also* ascites, cardiac failure, cirrhosis, effusion, glomerulonephritis, paracentesis, succussion

EAR, *see also* audiogram, audiology, audiometer, auditory, aural, cochlea, concha, Eustachian, fenestration, hypacusia, labyrinth, meatus, membrane (tympanic), myringitis, myringodectomy, myringotome, myringotomy, otic, otitis, otolaryngologist, otolaryngology, otologist, otosclerosis, otoscope, paracusia, stapes, tinnitus, tophus

EDEMA, *see also* cardiac failure, chilblain, bleb, blister, eczema, elephantiasis, hives, hydrarthrosis, hydrocele, hydrocephaly, hydrothorax, myxedema, pemphigus, phlyctenule, polyhydramnios, pericarditis, succussion, urticaria, wheal

Embolism, *see* embolus

EMBOLUS, *see also* heparin, infarct, phlebitis

ENDOCRINE, *see also* acetylcholine, acromegaly, ACTH, Addison's disease, adrenal gland, adrenalin, calcinosis, choline, cholinesterase, cortex, cortisone, cretinism, decalcification, denigration, endocrinopathy, estrogen, eunuchoidism, gigantism, gland, goiter, gonad, gonadotrophin, gynandromorphism, gynecomastia, hormone, hyperinsulinism, hyperpituitarism, hyperthyroidism, hypophysis, hypopituitarism, hypothyroidism, ketosteroid, masculinization, menarche, menopause, menses, menstruation, myxedema, orchis, ovary, ovulation, pancreas, parathyroid, pineal gland, pituitary, progeria, puberty, puerperium, sterility, struma, testis, testosterone, thymus, thyroid, thyrotoxicosis, thyroxin, virilism

EXANTHEMA, *see also* chicken pox, erysipelas, German measles, (rubella) measles, rickettsialpox, scarlet fever, smallpox, typhoid, typhus, varicella, variola

FEVER, *see also* afebrile, antipyretic, blackwater fever, brucellosis, carbuncle, cholera, coccidioidomycosis, common cold, dengue, diphtheria, exanthema, gout, hepatitis, influenza, kala azar, malaria, measles, mononucleosis, mumps, paratyphoid, peritonitis, plague, pneumonia, poliomyelitis, psittacosis, relapsing fever, rheumatism, rickettsialpox, Rocky Mountain spotted fever, rubeola, sarcoidosis, scarlet fever, sepsis, sleeping sickness, smallpox, trypanosomiasis, tsutsugamushi disease, tuberculosis, tularemia, typhoid, typhus, undulant fever, whooping cough, yellow fever

FINGER, *see also* anomaly, dactylitis, dactylus, felon, finger cot, phalanx, Raynaud's disease, syndactylus, thumb, whitlow

FUNGUS, *see also* fungicide, fungoid, mycology, mycosis, Oidium, Trichophyton

GALL BLADDER, *see also* abdomen, achalasia, bile, calculus, cholagogue, cholecystectomy, cholecystitis, cholecystogram, cholelith, cholesterol, colic, cyst, cystectomy, empyema, icteric, icterus, jaundice, laparotomy

Gas, *see* emphysema, flatulence, flatus, insufflation, vesicant

GENITALIA, *see also* anorchism, balanitis, balanus, bartholinitis, chancre, chancroid, chordee, clitoris, clitorism, coitus, colpalgia, colpectomy, colpaltitis, colpocele, colpoplasty, colpotomy, cremaster, cryptorchidectomy, cryptorchidopexy, cryptorchism, defloration, emasculation, epididymus, epididymectomy, epididymitis, episiotomy, epispadias, erection, erotogenic zones, eunuch, fellatio, fornication, frenulum, funiculitis, azoospermia, glans, gleet, gonad, gonadotrophin, gonorrhea, gynandromorphism, gynatresia, gynecologist, gynoplasty, hermaphrodite, hydrocele, hymen, hymenectomy, hymenotomy, hypospadias, hysterectomy, hysterosalpingectomy, imperforate, insemination, intrauterine, involution, jockey strap, kraurosis, labium, masturbation, meatus, menses, menstruation, metrorrhagia, mons pubis, mumps, nidation, nymphectomy, onanism, oophorectomy, oophoritis, orchiectomy, orchiopexy, orchis, orchitis, orgasm, os, ostium, ovarian, ovariectomy, ovary, oviduct, ovulation, ovum, panhysterectomy, parametritis, parametrium, paraspadias, patulous, penis, perineum, pessary, phallus, phimosis, placenta, potency, prepuce, priapism, prolapse, prostate, prostatectomy, prostatitis, pruritus vulvae, pseudohermaphrodite, puberty, pubes, puerperium, salpingectomy, salpingitis, salpingo-oophoritis, scrotum, semen, semination, smegma, sperm, spot (genital), syphilis, testes, testosterone, trichomonas, triorchid, urethra, urethritis, urogenital, urologist, urology, uterine, uterography, uterus, vagina, vaginismus, vaginitis, varicocele, vasectomy, vasotomy, venereal, virilism, vulva, vulvectomy, vulvitis, vulvovaginitis, womb

GIGANTISM, *see also* acromegaly, endocrinopathy, hyperpituitarism

GLAND, *see also* adenitis, adenoid, adenoma, adenopathy, adrenal gland, breast, endocrinology, endocrinopathy, mamma, mucous, mucus, ovary, pancreas, parathyroid, parotid, pineal gland, pituitary, prostate, thymus, thyroid

GLUCOSE, *see also* bronze diabetes, diabetes, glycosuria, hemochromatosis, hyperglycemia, hypoglycemia, test (glucose tolerance; Benedict's), tolerance (sugar), xanthoma

GOITER, *see also* albuminuria, goitrogenic, hemithyroidectomy, hyperthyroidism, hypothyroidism, infantilism, struma, thyroid, thyroxin, thyroidectomy

GONORRHEA, *see also* adenopathy, bubo, chordee, gleet, gonococcus, Neisseria, rheumatism, specific, urethritis, venereal

GOUT, *see also* hallux, podagra, tophus

"Grey matter," *see* cortex

Gullet, *see* diverticulum, esophagitis, esophagoscope, esophagus, gavage, heartburn, mediastinum, membrane, pharynx, stricture, thorax

HEAD, *see also* caput, cephalalgia, cephalic, contre-coup, cranium, fontanel, headache, microcephaly, migraine, neck, occipital, occiput, skull, temple, trephine, vertex, vertical

Hearing, *see* agnosia, audiogram, audiology, audiometer, auditory, aural, cochlea, ear, hypacusia, paracusia

HEART, *see also* albuminuria, aneurysm, angina (pectoris), anomaly, arrhythmia, ascites, ballistocardiogram, blood pressure, bradycardia, bruit, cardiac, cardiac failure, cardiology, coronary, decompensation, dextrocardia, diastole, digitalis, digitalization, dropsy, edema, effusion, electrocardiogram, empyema, endocarditis, extrasystole, fibrillation, flutter, heartblock, heart murmur, heart rate, heart sound, hemopericardium, massage, mitral, murmur, muscle, myocarditis, myocardium, necrosis, palpitation, pancarditis, paracentesis (of pericardium), pericardiectomy, pericarditis, pericardium, phonocardiography, presystolic, syncope, systole, tachycardia, tamponade, thrill, valve, valvulitis, valvulotomy

Heel, *see* Achilles, calcaneus, disc, os ^{2}, sciatica

HERNIA, *see also* hernioplasty, incarceration, inguinal, rupture, sac, strangulation

HOMOSEXUALITY, *see also* dionism, hermaphrodite, inversion, lesbianism, metamorphosis, oral erotism, pederasty, pseudohermaphrodite, sapphism, sodomy, virilism

HORMONE, *see also* acetylcholine, ACTH, adrenal gland, adrenalin, choline, cholinesterase, cortisone, endocrine, endocrinology, estrogen, gonadotrophin, ketosteroid, thyroxin

ICTERUS, *see also* hepatitis, anemia, jaundice, liver, yellow fever

Indigestion, *see* altitude sickness, biliousness

INFECTION, *see also* acid-fast, antibiotic, antibody, antigen, antisepsis, antitoxin, asepsis, bacillemia, bacillus, bacitracin, bacteremia, bactericide, bacteriophage, bacteriostasis, bacterium, carbuncle, chemotherapy, disinfectant, furuncle, furunculosis, hordeolum, immune, immunity, immunology, microbe, purulent, pus, pustule, pyoderma, reinfection, runaround, sepsis, septicemia, suppuration, whitlow

INTELLIGENCE QUOTIENT, *see also* cretinism, dementia, epicanthus, idiocy, imbecility, infantilism, mongolism, moron, myxedema

IRIS, *see also* dyscoria, iridectomy, iridocyclitis, iridocystectomy, iritis, iritoectomy, keratoiritis, midriasis, myosis, synechia

KETOSTEROID, *see also* ACTH, cortisone, gonadotrophin, hormone, testosterone

KIDNEY, *see also* abdomen, albuminuria, ascites, calculus, capsule, cortex, cystoscope, decompensation, dropsy, ectopia, floating, genitourinary, glomerulonephritis, glomerulus, gout, gravel, hematuria, hypernephroma, lithiasis, nephrectomy, nephritis, nephrolithiasis, nephrolithotomy, nephroma, nephropexy, nephrosilerosis, nephrosis, nephrotomy, parenchyma, perinephric, purpura (symptomatic), pyelitis, pyelogram, pyelonephritis, pyuria, ureter, ureterolith, ureterotomy, urogenital, urologist, urology

LARYNX, *see also* aphonia, croup, epiglottis, laryngectomy, laryngismus, laryngitis, laryngoscope, laryngotomy, mutism, stertor, trachea

LENS, *see also* aphakia, astigmatism, cataract, lenticular, needling, opacity, presbyopia, vitreous

LEUKEMIA, *see also* dyscrasia, leukoblast, leukocyte, leukocytosis, leukopenia, lymphadenopathy, lymphoblastoma, priapism

LEUKOCYTE, *see also* agranulocytosis, anemia, blood count, corpuscle, eosinophile, granulocyte, leukoblast, leukocytolysis, leukocytosis, leukemia, leukopenia, lymphocyte, monocyte, mononucleosis, neutrophil, phagocyte

LIVER, *see also* abdomen, ascites, bile, bronze diabetes, capsule, chloasma, cholagogue, cholangitis, cholelith, cholemia, choluria, cirrhosis, dropsy, duct, endamoeba, gall bladder, hemochromatosis, heparin, hepatitis, hepatomegaly, hydatid, icterus, jaundice, kala azar, lobe, parenchyma, schistomiasis, yellow fever

LUNG, *see also* ascariasis, aspergillosis, acid-fast, asthma, Ayerza's syndrome, bagassosis, beryllosis, blast injury, bronchiole, bronchiolitis, bronchitis, bronchogenic, bronchogram, bronchography, bronchopneumonia, bronchoscope, bronchospasm, bronchostenosis, bronchus, byssinosis, calcicosis, coccidioidomycosis, dyspnea, echinococcosis, emphysema, empyema, influenza, iron lung, lobe, lobectomy, lobule, moniliasis, necatoriasis, occupational disease, oleothorax, ornithosis, parenchyma, phthisiology, phthisis, pneumonectomy, pneumonia, pneumonoconiosis, pneumothorax, psittacosis, rale, respiration, resuscitation, rhonchus, sarcoidosis, siderosis, silicosis, succussion, thorax, tuberculosis, wheeze

MENSES, *see also* amenorrhea, climacteric, dysmenorrhea, emmenagogue, menarche, menhidrosis, menopause, menorrhagia, menorrhea, menstruation, pain (intermenstrual), puberty

METABOLISM, *see also* anabolism, catabolism, cretinism, gout, hyperthyroidism, hypothyroidism, ketosis, maize, marasmus, myxedema, nephrosis, nutrition, obesity, pellagra, xanthoma

Miscarriage, *see* abortion

MOUTH, *see also* ariboflavinosis, canker, cheilosis, denture, edentate, endamoeba (gingivalis), gingiva, gingivitis, glossa, glossalgia, glossodynia, glossopyrosis, glossotrichia, harelip, hemiglossectomy, herpes, jaw, angina (agranulo), lingua, lumpy jaw, mandible, mastication, maxilla, microglossia, mumps, oral, oral erotism, os[1], ostium, palate, palatoplegia, ptyalin, ramus, saliva, salivation, sialorrhea, sprue, stomatitis, thrush, tongue, uvula, vestibule

MUSCLE, *see also* abasia, abduct, amyotonia, atony, barbiturism, biceps, buttock, catalepsy, cataplexy, chorea, claudication, clonus, contracture, convulsion, cramp, creatine, creatinine, curare, deltoid, diaphragm, diplegia, dystrophy, fibrillation, gastrocnemius, gelotolepsy, hemiplegia, heterophoria, kinesthesia, lameness, locomotion, monoplegia, myalgia, myasthenia, myatonia, myocardium, myoclonus, myoma, myositis, myotoma, obturator, oculomotor, ophthalmoplegia, palatoplegia, palsy, paralysis, paraplegia, paresis, pectoral, phrenoplegia, platysma, psoas, ptosis, quadriceps, quadriplegia, rhomboideus, rigidity, St. Vitus' dance, scalenus, sclerosis, spasm, thenar, tic, trapezius

Mustard plaster, *see* counter irritant

MYCOSIS, *see also* actinomycosis, aspergillosis, blastomycosis, coccidioidomycosis, dermatophytosis, dermatophytid, epidermophytid, epidermophytosis, favus, fungicide, fungus, jungle rot, moniliasis, mycology, necatoriasis, Oidium, stomatitis, thrush, tinea, Trichophyton, trichophytosis

MYXEDEMA, *see also* endocrinopathy, hypothyroidism, obesity, thyroid

NAIL, *see also* dystrophy mediona canaliformis, nail biting, onychia, onychomycosis, onychophagia, onyx, pachyonychia, paronychia, perionychia, runaround

Nembutal, *see* barbiturism

NERVOUS SYSTEM, *see also* acetylcholine, alogia, amblyopia, amyotonia, analgesia, anesthesia, anodyne, aphasia, apoplexy, apraxia, arachnoid, autonomic, beriberi, bulimia, causalgia, cerebellum, cerebration, cerebrum, choline, chorea, cochlea, coma, convulsion, cortex, cranium, curare, dementia, diplegia, disorientation, dura mater, dyskinesia, encephalitis, encephalogram, encephalomalacia, engram, epilepsy, ganglion, glioma, hemianesthesia, hemianopsia, hemiplegia, hydrocephaly, hypesthesia, infantile paralysis, innervation, intelligence quotient, kinesthesia, lead poisoning, leprosy, lobotomy, medulla, meninges, meningioma, meningism, meningitides, meningitis, monoplegia, myelin, myelitis, myelogram, narcolepsy, nerve, neuralgia, neuritis, neurofibromatosis, neurologist, neuron, neuropathy, neuroretinitis, pachymeningitis, pain (girdle; referred), palsy, paralysis, paraplegia, parasympathetic, paresis, paresthesia, phrenic, pia mater, pilomotor, pneumoencephalography, poliomyelitis, quadriplegia, rabies, reflex, saturnism, sciatica, sclerosis, sleeping sickness, stroke, sympathectomy, syringomyelia, tabes, thalamus, trypanosomiasis, uncinate fit, vagus, vasomotor

Niacin, *see* maize

NOSE, *see also* ala, anosmia, common cold, coryza, hay fever, June cold, naris, nasopharynx, nasus, paranasal, philtrum, polyp, postnasal, ragweed, rhinitis, rhinologist, rhinology, rhinophyma, rhinorrhaphy, rhinoscleroma, rose fever, septum, sinus, spot (genital), vomer

Nosebleed, *see* epistaxis

OCCUPATIONAL DISEASE, *see also* anthracosis, anthrax, asbestosis, bagassosis, beryllosis, byssinosis, calcicosis, lead poisoning, palsy, pneumonoconiosis, siderosis, silicosis, tennis arm

ORGASM, *see also* autoerotism, coitus, ejaculatio, ejaculation, end pleasure, erotogenic, erotogenic zones, erotomania, flagellation, forepleasure, fornication, frottage, genital, genitalia, gonad, idiogamist, impotence, insemination, libido, masturbation, onanism, semination, semen

PANCREAS, *see also* achylia (pancreatica), catalyst, gland, hyperinsulinism, pancreatine, pancreatitis

PARATHYROID, *see also* calcinosis, decalcification, endocrine, endocrinology, endocrinopath, gland, hormone, secretion

Penicillin, *see* allergy, antibiotic

PENIS, *see also* balanitis, balanus, cantharides, chancre, chordee, coitus, condom, epispadias, erection, eunuch, fellatio, fellator, fellatrice, genitalia, glans, gleet, hypospadias, paraspadias, phallus, phimosis, prepuce, priapism, saltpeter, smegma

Perspiration, *see* accommodation, antipyretic, bromhidrosis, sunstroke
PHARYNX, *see also* diphtheria, douche, dysphagia, epiglottis, globus, glot-
    tis, hay fever, lead poisoning, nasopharynx, oropharynx, pharyngec-
    tomy, pharyngitis, pharyngoscope, retropharynx
Phenobarbital, *see* barbiturism, luminal
PHOBIA, *see also* acrophobia, agoraphobia, cardiophobia, dextrophobia,
    ergophobia, galeophobia, hydrophobia, photophobia
Pimple(s), *see* acne, ecthyma, eczema, papilla, papulopustular, sycosis
PINEAL GLAND, *see also* endocrine, endocrinology, endocrinopathy, hor-
    mone
PITUITARY, *see also* acromegaly, ACTH, endocrine, gigantism, gland,
    hormone, hyperpituitarism, hypopituitarism, infantilism, progeria,
    sella
PLACENTA, *see also* afterbirth, chorion, abortion, curette, curettage,
    decidua, intrauterine
PNEUMONOCONIOSIS, *see also* anthracosis, asbestosis, bagassosis, beryllo-
    sis, byssinosis, calcicosis, siderosis, silicosis
PNEUMOTHORAX, *see also* phthisiology, phthisis
PROSTATE, *see also* capsule, gonorrhea, prostatectomy, prostatitis
Purgative, *see* aperient, calomel

Rheumatic fever, *see* adventitious, rheumatism, aortitis, pericarditis,
    stenosis
Riboflavin, *see* ariboflavinosis, cheilosis
RUPTURE, *see also* hernia, strangulation

Scab, *see* incrustation, variolation
Scalp, *see* acromegaly, dandruff, epicranium
Scar, *see* cicatrix, umbilicus
Sensitivity, *see* allergy, desensitization
SERUM, *see also* blood typing, bovine, effusion, hematocrit, hematology,
    hemoglobinemia, immunity, intoxication, plasma, test
SIGMOID, *see also* barium sulfate, colic, colon, diverticulum, dysentery,
    Hirshsprung's disease, intestine, sigmoidectomy, sigmoidoscope
SINUS, *see also* antrum, ethmoid, ethmoidectomy, ethmoiditis, pansinu-
    sitis, paranasal, sinusitis, sphenoid, sphenoiditis, turbinate
Smell, *see* anosmia
Sodium bicarbonate, *see* acidosis, alkalosis
Sour stomach, *see* acidity
SPERM, *see also* aspermatism, azoospermia, ejaculatio, emission, insemi-
    nation, onanism, orgasm, semen, spermatocidal, spermatozoa
SPINE, *see also* atlas, disc, joint, kyphosis, lordosis, lumbosacral, punc-

ture (lumbar), sacroiliac, sacrum, scoliosis, spina, spondylalgia, spondylitis, vertebra

SPIROCHETE, *see also* aneurysm, chancre, granuloma, gumma, osteitis, rhagades, stigma, syphilis, test, yaws

SPLEEN, *see also* abdomen, ague, jaundice, laparotomy, leukemia, lymphoblastoma, malaria, splenectomy, splenomegaly

STOMACH, *see also* abdomen, achalasia, achlorhydria, achylia, acidity, alimentary, anemia, annulus, autodigestion, barium sulfate, canker, cardiospasm, chyme, diverticulum, dyspepsia, fistula, gastralgia, gastectomy, gastric, gastritis, gastroenteritis, gastroenterologist, gastroenterostomy, gastrojejunostomy, gastrorrhagia, gavage, heartburn, juice, nausea, pyloroplasty, pylorus, stenosis, ulcer

Suffocation, *see* angina, asphyxia, cyanosis

Sugar, *see* adrenalin, bronze diabetes, carbohydrate, diabetes mellitus, glucose, glycosuria, hyperglycemia, hyperinsulinism, hypoglycemia, lactose, liver, placebo, sweat, test, tolerance, urine

Terramycin, *see* antibiotic

TESTIS, *see also* anorchism, cremaster, cryptorchidectomy, cryptorchidopexy, cryptorchism, emasculation, epididymectomy, epididymis, epididymitis, eunuch, eunuchoidism, funiculitis, genital, genitourinary, gonad, gonadotrophin, hydrocele, jockey strap, mumps, orchic, orchiectomy, orchiopexy, orchis, orchitis, scrotum, testosterone, triorchid

THORAX, *see also* costalgia, costectomy, effusion, empyema, gibbous, hemothorax, hydrothorax, kyphosis, lung, heart, mediastinum, pectoral, pectus, pleura, pleurisy, pleurodynia, pneumothorax, rib, thoracectomy, thoracentesis, thoracoplasty

THYROID, *see also* cretinism, endocrinology, endocrine, endocrinopathy, flush, goiter, goitrogenic, hormone, hyperthyroidism, hypothyroidism, isthmus, myxedema, struma, thyroiditis, thyroidectomy, thyrotoxicosis, thyroxin

TOE, *see also* bunion, dacylitis, dactylus, erythromelalgia, gout, hallux, hammertoe, metatarsalgia, phalanx, podagra

TONGUE, *see also* frenulum, glossa, glossalgia, glossectomy, glossitis, glossodynia, glossopyrosis, glossotrichia, hemiglosectomy, hypoglossal, lingua, papilla (gustatory)

TONSIL, *see also* adenoid, adenoidectomy, atrophy, fauces, paratonsillar, peritonsillar, quinsy, snare, tonsillectomy

TRACHEA, *see also* death rattle, hemoptysis, tracheitis, tracheotomy

TUMOR, *see also* adenoma, cancer, cancroid, carcinoma, chondroma, condyloma, cyst, dermoid, echinococcosis, epithelioma, excrescence, exostosis, fibroma, ganglion, goiter, granuloma, gumma, hemangioma, hematoma, hydatid, hepatoma, hypernephroma, keloid, leiomyoma, leiomyosarcoma, lipoma, liposarcoma, lymphadenoma, lymphadenopathy, lymphoblastoma, melanoma, meningioma, myeloma, myoma, neoplasm, nephroma, odontoma, onocology, osteocarcinoma, osteoma, osteochondroma, papilloma, paraffinoma, rhabdomyoma, rhinoscleroma, sarcoma, teratoma, tumescence, wen

ULCER, *see also* bed sore, chancroid, chancre, decubitus, excoriation, ulceration

UMBILICUS, *see also* areola (umbilical), hypogastrium, omphalitis, omphalos

URETER, *see also* calculus, colic, cystoscope, obstruction, pyelogram, pyelonephritis, ureterolith, ureterotomy

URETHRA, *see also* bougie, catheter, cystoscope, gonorrhea, meatus, stricture, urethritis

URINE, *see also* albuminuria, anuria, bacteriuria, biliuria, bronze diabetes, choluria, creatinine, diabetes, diuresis, dysuria, emiction, enuresis, genitourinary, glucose, glycosuria, gravel, hematuria, hemochromatosis, hemoglobinuria, incontinence, kidney, nephrosis, nocturia, paracentesis (of bladder), polyuria, pyelitis, pyelonephritis, ureter, urethra, urethritis, urogenital, urology, urologist

UTERUS, *see also* abortion, afterbirth, anteversion, cervicectomy, cervicitis, cervix, chorion, decidua, endometriosis, endometrium, estrus, feticide, hysterectomy, hysterosalpingectomy, intrauterine, involution, labor, malposition, metrorrhagia, nidation, pain (after; bearing down), panhysterectomy, parametritis, parametrium, placenta, prolapse, puerperium, uterine, uterography, womb

VAGINA, *see also* balanitis, balanus, bartholinitis, clitoris, clitorism, coitus, colpalgia, colpectomy, colpaltitis, colpoplasty, colpotomy, defloration, diaphragm, episiotomy, erection, flatus, genitalia, glans, hymen, hymenectomy, hymenotomy, introitus, labium, prepuce, smegma, vaginismus, vaginitis, vulva, vulvovaginitis

VEIN, *see also* basilic vein, hemorrhoid, jugular, phlebitis, phlebolith, phlebosclerosis, phlebothrombosis, phlebotomy, saphenous vein, thromboangiitis, thrombophlebitis, varicose

VERTEBRA, *see also* atlas, gibbous, humpback, kyphosis, lumbosacral, lumbar, myelogram, radicular, radiculitis, sacroiliac, sacrum, scoliosis, spine, spondylalgia, spondylitis

VIRUS, *see also* Australian X disease, common cold, dengue, encephalitis, German measles, hepatitis (infectious), herpes, hydrophobia, influenza, keratoconjunctivitis (epidemic), measles, meningitis, mumps,

TABLE OF CALORIES
IN AVERAGE PORTION OF FOOD

NAME	AVERAGE PORTION		
	Measure	Wt./Gms	Calories
DAIRY PRODUCTS			
Butter	1 tbsp.	14	100
Buttermilk	1 cup	244	86
Cheese			
Blue mold	1 oz.	28	104
Cheddar	1 oz.	28	113
Cottage	1 oz.	28	27
Cream	1 oz.	28	106
Swiss	1 oz.	28	105
Cream, light	1 tbsp.	15	30
whipping	1 tbsp.	15	50
Ice Cream, plain	1 slice	81	167
Milk, cow			
Fluid, whole	1 cup	244	166
Fluid, non-fat	1 cup	246	87
Evaporated	1 cup	252	346
Non-fat solids, dry	1 tbsp.	8	28
Malted, beverage	1 cup	270	281
Chocolate flavor	1 cup	250	185
Milk, goat, liquid	1 cup	244	164
Sherbet	1/2 cup	96	118
FATS, OILS, and SHORTENINGS			
Butter	1 tbsp.	14	100
Fats, vegetable, cooking	1 cup	200	1768
Margarine	1 cup	14	126
Mayonnaise	1 tbsp.	14	100
Oils, salad, cooking	1 tbsp.	13	92

The tables on these pages were adapted from Tables of Food
Composition in Nutritional Data published by H.J. Heinz Company and reproduced with the permission of the publishers.

NAME	AVERAGE PORTION		
	Measure	Wt./Gms	Calories

FATS, OILS, and SHORTENINGS

Salt pork fat	2 oz.	60	470
Salad dressing, French	1 tbsp.	15	60

FRUITS

BERRIES

Blackberries, raw	1 cup	144	82
Blueberries, raw	1 cup	140	85
Blueberries, cnd., swt.	1 cup	249	245
Cranberries, raw	1 cup	113	54
Cranberry sauce, cnd., swt.	1 cup	277	550
Currants, red, raw	1/2 cup	55	30
Gooseberries	1 cup	150	59
Loganberries, raw	1 cup	144	90
Raspberries, blk., raw	1 cup	134	100
Raspberries, red, raw	1 cup	123	70
Raspberries, red, frz.	3 oz.	86	84
Strawberries, raw	1 cup	149	54
Strawberries, frz.	3 oz.	86	82

CITRUS FRUIT

Grapefruit, raw	1 cup sections	194	77
Grapefruit, cnd., swt.	1 cup	249	181
Lemon	1, 2" diam.	100	20
Lime	1, 1 1/2" long	68	19
Orange	1 med. 3" diam.	215	70
Tangerine	1 med. 2 1/2" diam.	114	35

NAME	AVERAGE PORTION		
	Measure	Wt./Gms	Calories

FRUITS

MELONS

Cantaloupe	1/2 melon, 5" diam.	385	37
Honey dew	1, 2'x7" wedge	150	49
Watermelon	1/2 sl., 3/4 x 10"	345	45

TREE, VINE and OTHER FRUITS

Apple, raw	1 med. 2 1/2" diam.	150	76
Apple, dry, unckd.	1 cup	114	315
Apricot, raw	3 apricots	114	54
Apricot, cnd., swt.	4 med. 1/2's, 2 tbsp.	122	97
Apricot, dry	40 1/2's	150	393
Apricot, frz.	3 oz.	84	81
Avocado	1/2, 3 1/2 x 3 1/4"	114	280
Banana	1 med. 6x11 1/2"	150	88
Cherry, raw	1 cup, pitted	154	94
Cherry, red, sour, cnd.	1 cup, pitted	254	122
Date, dried	1 cup, pitted	177	505
Fig, cnd., swt.	3, 2 tbsp. syrup	115	130
Fig, dried	1 large, 1x2"	21	57

NAME	AVERAGE PORTION		
	Measure	Wt./Gms	Calories

TREE, VINE and OTHER FRUITS

NAME	Measure	Wt./Gms	Calories
Grapes, raw			
American slip skin	1 cup	153	84
European adherent	1 cup		
	40 grapes	160	102
Guava, raw	1 small	80	49
Peach, raw	1 med.		
	2x2 1/2"		
	diam.	114	45
Peach, cnd., swt.	1 cup	258	175
Peach, frz., swt.	4 oz.	112	99
Peach, dry, unckd.	1 cup	160	424
Pear, raw	1, 3x2 1/2"		
	diam.	182	95
Pear, cnd., swt.	2 1/2's,		
	2 tbsp.		
	syrup	117	80
Plum, raw	1, 2" diam.	60	30
Plum, cnd., swt.	1 cup	256	186
Prune, dry	4 large		
	prunes	40	94
Raisin, dry	1 cup	160	430
Rhubarb, frz.	1 cup	273	202

FRUIT JUICES and OTHER FRUIT PRODUCTS

NAME	Measure	Wt./Gms	Calories
Apple juice, frz./cnd.	1 cup	249	124
Apple sauce, frz./cnd., swt.	1 cup	254	185
Apricot nectar	1 cup	254	170
Fruit cocktail, cnd., swt.	1 cup	257	180
Grape juice, cnd., swt.	6 oz.	180	120
Grapefruit juice, cnd., swt.	1 cup	251	131
Lemon juice, cnd.	1 tbsp.	15	4

NAME   AVERAGE PORTION

                            Measure   Wt./Gms   Calories

FRUIT JUICES and OTHER FRUIT PRODUCTS

Name	Measure	Wt./Gms	Calories
Lime juice, fresh	1 cup	246	57
Olives, green	10, mammoth	65	72
Olives, ripe, Mission	10, mammoth	65	106
Orange juice, fresh	1 cup	246	108
Orange juice, cnd.	1 cup	251	135
Orange & grapefruit juice, cnd., swt.	1 cup	251	132
Pineapple juice, cnd.	1 cup	249	121
Prune juice, cnd.	1 cup	240	170
Tangerine juice, cnd.	1 cup	246	95
Tomato juice, cnd.	1 cup	242	50

GRAINS and GRAIN PRODUCTS

Breakfast Cereals

Name	Measure	Wt./Gms	Calories
Bran flakes	1 cup	40	117
Corn flakes	1 cup	25	96
Farina, ckd.	1 cup	238	105
Oat bkfst. cereal	1 cup	25	100
Oatmeal, ckd.	1 cup	238	150
Puffed rice	1 cup	14	55
Puffed wheat	1 cup	12	43
Rice flakes	1 cup	30	117
Wheat flakes	1 cup	35	125
Wheat, whole, meal	1/4 cup	30	103

FLOURS, MEALS and OTHER FARINACEOUS MATERIALS

Name	Measure	Wt./Gms	Calories
Barley, pearled, light	1 cup	204	710
Buckwheat flour, light	1 cup	98	342
Corn grits, ckd.	1 cup	242	122

NAME

AVERAGE PORTION

	Measure	Wt./Gms	Calories

FLOURS, MEALS and OTHER FARINACEOUS MATERIALS

Name	Measure	Wt./Gms	Calories
Corn meal, whole	1 cup	127	459
Corn meal, degermed	1 cup	145	527
Farina	1 cup	169	625
Flour, rye, dark	1 cup	80	285
Flour, wheat, 80%	1 cup	110	400
Flour, wheat, self-rising	1 cup	110	384
Flour, wheat, all-purpose	1 cup	110	400
Flour, wheat, cake	1 cup	100	364
Rice, brown	1 cup	208	748
Rice, converted	1 cup	187	677
Rice, white	1 cup	191	692
Starch, pure	1 tbsp.	8	29
Tapioca, dry	1 cup	152	547
Wild rice	1 cup	163	593
Wheat germ	1 cup	68	246

BAKED and COOKED PRODUCTS

BREADS

Name	Measure	Wt./Gms	Calories
Boston Brown	1 3/4" slice	48	105
Cracked wheat	1 1/2" slice	23	60
French or Vienna	1 pound	453	1225
Raisin	1 1/2" slice	23	65
Rye (1/3 rye flour)	1 1/2" slice	23	57
White, 4% non-fat milk solids	1 1/2" slice	23	63

NAME	AVERAGE PORTION		
	Measure	Wt./Gms	Calories

BAKED and COOKED PRODUCTS

BREADS

Whole wheat	1 1/2" slice	23	55
Bread crumbs, dry	1 cup	88	339

CAKES

Angel food	2" sec. of 8" cake	41	110
Foundation	1 sq. 3x 2x1 3/4"	66	230
Fruit, dark	2x2x1/2"	30	106
Plain	1 2 3/4" cupcake	50	161
Sponge	2" sec. of 8" cake	40	117

Corn bread	1 2 3/4" muffin	48	103
Crackers, graham	2 medium	14	55
Crackers, saltines	2, 2" square	8	34
Custard, baked	1 cup	248	283
Doughnuts	1	32	136
Fig bars	1, large	25	87
Gingerbread	1, 2" cube	55	180
Macaroni, dry	1 cup	123	463
Macaroni & cheese, ckd.	1 cup	220	464
Muffins	1, 2 3/4" muffin	48	135
Noodles, egg, ckd.	1 cup	60	107
Pancakes, wheat	1, 4" diam.	27	60
Pancakes, buckwheat	1, 4" diam.	27	48

NAME	AVERAGE PORTION		
	Measure	Wt./Gms	Calories

BAKED and COOKED PRODUCTS

PIES

Apple	1, 4" sector of 9" diam. pie	220	330
Mince	"	135	340
Pumpkin	"	131	265
Pretzel	5 small sticks	5	18
Rolls, plain	1, 1/12 lb.	39	120
Rolls, sweet	1 roll	55	178
Rye wafers	2 wafers	13	43
Spaghetti, ckd.	1 cup	148	220
Waffles	1, 4 1/2x 5 5/8x1/2"	75	216

NUTS and NUT PRODUCTS

Almonds, dry	1 cup	140	850
Brazil, nuts, shelled	1 cup	140	905
Cashews, roasted	1 cup	140	810
Chestnuts, fresh	20	50	95
Coconut, dry, swt.	1 cup shreds	62	344
Peanuts, roasted	1 cup	144	805
Peanut butter	1 tbsp.	16	92
Pecans, raw	1 cup of 1/2's	108	752
Walnuts, Eng., raw	1 cup 1/2's	100	654

NAME	AVERAGE PORTION		
	Measure	Wt./Gms	Calories

MEAT, POULTRY, and SEAFOOD

BEEF

Chuck, ckd.	3 oz.	86	265
Hamburger, ckd.	3 oz. ground	86	316
Porterhouse, ckd.	3 oz.	86	293
Rib roast, ckd.	3 oz.	86	266
Round, ckd.	3 oz.	86	197
Corn beef, cnd.	3 oz.	86	180
Corn beef hash, cnd.	3 oz.	86	120
Dried or chipped beef	2 oz.	56	115
Roast beef, cnd.	3 oz.	86	189

LAMB

Med. fat, raw	3 oz.	86	273
Rib chop, raw	4 oz.	115	409
Rib chop, ckd.	4 oz.	115	480
Leg roast, raw	3 oz.	86	202
Leg roast, ckd.	3 oz.	86	314

PORK

Bacon, fried	2 slices	16	97
Bacon, Canadian, raw	4 oz.	115	262
Ham, fresh, raw	3 oz.	86	296
Ham, cured, ckd.	3 oz.	86	340
Pork, luncheon meat, cnd.	2 oz.	57	165

VEAL

Veal, med., fat	4 oz.	115	219
Veal, cutlet, ckd.	3 oz.	86	184
Stew meat, ckd.	3 oz.	86	252

NAME	AVERAGE PORTION		
	Measure	Wt./Gms	Calories

VARIETY MEATS and MIXTURES

NAME	Measure	Wt./Gms	Calories
Brains	3 oz.	86	106
Chile con carne	1/3 cup	85	170
Heart, beef, raw	3 oz.	86	92
Kidneys, beef, raw	3 oz.	86	120
Liver, beef, raw	3 oz.	86	117
Liver, beef, fried	2 oz.	57	118
Liver, calf, raw	3 oz.	86	121
Liver, pork, raw	3 oz.	86	115
Sausage, bologna	1x1 1/2" diam.	211	467
Sausage, frankfurter, ckd.	1, 7x3/4"	51	124
Sausage, liverwurst	2 oz.	57	150
Sausage, pork, raw	2, 3 1/2" long	55	158
Tongue, beef	4 oz.	115	235

FISH and SHELL FISH

NAME	Measure	Wt./Gms	Calories
Bluefish, baked	4 oz.	115	178
Clams, raw	4 oz.	115	92
Cod, raw	4 oz.	115	85
Cod, dried	1 oz.	28	106
Crabs, cnd. or ckd.	3 oz.	86	90
Flounder, raw	4 oz.	115	78
Frog legs, raw	4 oz.	115	82
Haddock, ckd.	1 fillet, 4x3x1/2"	100	158
Halibut, raw	4 oz.	115	145
Halibut, ckd.	1 fillet, 4x3x1/2"	126	230
Herring, raw	1 small herring	100	191

NAME	AVERAGE PORTION		
	Measure	Wt./Gms	Calories

FISH and SHELL FISH

Herring, kippered	1 small herring	100	211
Lobster, raw	1/2 average	100	88
Lobster, cnd.	3 oz.	86	78
Mackerel, cnd.	3 oz.	86	155
Oysters, raw	1 cup, 13-19 med.	238	200
Oysters, stew	1 cup, 6-8 oysters	240	244
Salmon, raw	3 oz.	86	192
Salmon, cnd.	3 oz.	86	120
Sardines, cnd.	3 oz. drained	86	182
Pilchards, cnd.	3 oz.	86	171
Scallops, raw	4 oz.	115	90
Shad, raw	4 oz.	115	191
Shrimp, cnd.	3 oz.	86	110
Swordfish, ckd.	1 steak, 3x3x1/2"	125	223
Tuna fish, cnd.	3 oz. drained	86	170

EGGS and POULTRY

Chicken, fryers, raw	1 breast	224	210
Chicken, roasters, raw	4 oz.	115	227
Chicken, cnd.	3 oz.	86	169
Chicken liver	2 med. livers	75	106
Duck	4 oz.	115	370
Goose	4 oz.	115	420
Turkey	4 oz.	115	304

NAME	AVERAGE PORTION		
	Measure	Wt./Gms	Calories

EGGS and POULTRY

EGGS, RAW

White	1	31	15
Yolk	1 cup	17	61
Whole	1 medium	54	77

EGGS, DRIED

White	1 cup	56	223
Yolk	1 cup	96	666
Whole	1 cup	108	640

SUGARS and SWEETS

CANDIED PEEL

Citron	1 oz.	28	89
Ginger root	1 small piece	25	85
Lemon, orange or grapefruit	1 small piece	10	32
Butterscotch	3/4" sq. x 3/8"	5	20
Caramels	7/8" sq. x 1/2"	10	42
Chocolate, swtd., milk	3/4"x11/2 x 1/4"	6	30
Chocolate with almonds	"	6	32
Chocolate creams	1 1/4" dm. x 3/4"	14	55
Fondant	1" sq. x 5/8"	8	28

NAME   AVERAGE PORTION

                               Measure   Wt./Gms   Calories

SUGARS and SWEETS

Name	Measure	Wt./Gms	Calories
Fudge, plain	2" sq. x 5/8"	45	185
Hard candy	3, 3/4" dm.	8	31
Marshmallows	5, 1 1/4" dm.	30	98
Peanut brittle	1 1/2"x3"	15	66
Chocolate, bitter	3/4" x 1 1/2" x 1/4"	6	30
Chocolate, plain, swt.	same	6	28
Chocolate syrup	1 tbsp.	19	40
Cocoa, bkfst.	2 tbsp.	5	15
Cocoa, beverage, milk	1 cup	250	236
Honey	1 tbsp.	21	62
Jams, marmalades, etc.	1 tbsp.	20	55
Jellies	1 tbsp.	20	50
Molasses, cane, light	1 tbsp.	20	50
Molasses, cane, black	1 tbsp.	20	43
Syrup, table, blends	1 tbsp.	20	57
Sugar, cane or beet	1 tbsp.	12	48
Sugar, brown	1 tbsp.	14	51
Corn sugar	1 tbsp.	13	45
Maple sugar	piece 1-3/4x 1 1/4x1/2"	30	104

VEGETABLES, ROOTS and TUBERS

Name	Measure	Wt./Gms	Calories
Beets, ckd.	1 cup	165	68
same, cnd.	1 cup	246	82
Carrots, raw	1 cup, grated	110	45
Carrots, cnd.	1 cup, diced	145	44
Parsnips, ckd.	1 cup, diced	155	94
Potatoes, boiled	1, 5x2 1/2"	205	252
Same, candied	1, 6x1-3/4"	150	270

NAME   AVERAGE PORTION

                                        Measure   Wt./Gms   Calories

VEGETABLES, ROOTS and TUBERS

Name	Measure	Wt./Gms	Calories
Potatoes, baked	1 med. 2 1/2" in diam.	100	97
Same, boiled	1 med.	142	120
Radishes, raw	4 small	40	4
Rutabagas, ckd.	1 cup diced	155	50
Turnips, ckd.	1 cup	155	42

LEAF and STEM

Name	Measure	Wt./Gms	Calories
Asparagus, ckd.	1 cup cut spears	175	36
Asparagus, cnd.	6 med. spears	126	22
Beet greens, ckd.	1 cup	145	39
Brussel sprouts, ckd.	1 cup	130	60
Cabbage, raw	1 cup, shredded	100	24
Cabbage, ckd.	1 cup, diced	170	40
Sauerkraut, cnd.	1 cup, drained	150	32
Celery, raw	1 cup, diced	100	18
Chard, leaves, raw	1 1/2 cup	100	27
Chard, leaves, stalks, ckd.	1 cup	145	30
Chicory, French endive	1/4 sm. head	15	3
Chives	1 tbsp. chopped	7	4
Cress, water	1/2 cup	20	5
Endive, raw	1 lb.	460	90
Kale, raw	1 3/4 cup	175	70
Kohlrabi, raw	1 cup	138	41
Lettuce, headed	2 lg. or 4 sm. leaves	50	7
Mustard greens, ckd.	1 cup	140	31

NAME	AVERAGE PORTION		
	Measure	Wt./Gms	Calories

LEAF and STEM

Onions, mature, raw	1, 2 1/2" diam.	110	50
Onions, mature, ckd.	1 cup	210	79
Onions, young, green	6 small, less tops	50	23
Parsley	1 tbsp.	3 1/2	1
Spinach, ckd.	1 cup	80	46
Spinach, cnd.	1 cup	232	45
Turnip greens, ckd.	1 cup	145	43

FLOWER, FRUIT and SEED VEGETABLES

Artichoke	1, 3" diam.	50	33
Beans, red, kidney, cnd. or ckd.	1 cup	255	230
Beans, lima, green, ckd.	1 cup	160	152
Beans, lima, green, cnd.	1 cup	249	176
Beans, lima, dry	1 cup	183	610
Beans, snap, green, ckd.	1 cup	125	27
Beans, snap, green, cnd.	1 cup	125	27
Broccoli, ckd.	1 cup	150	44
Broccoli, frz.	1 cup	120	36
Cauliflower, ckd.	1 cup	120	30
Cauliflower, frz.	1 1/4 cup	125	27
Corn, swt., ckd.	1 ear, 5"	140	85
Corn, swt., cnd.	1 cup	116	140
Cucumbers, raw	6, 1/8" slices	50	6
Egg plant, raw	2 slices	250	60
Lentils, dry, split	1/4 cup	60	204
Mushrooms, cnd.	1 cup	244	28
Okra, ckd.	8 pods	85	28
Peas, green, ckd.	1 cup	60	111
Peas, green, cnd.	1 cup	60	145

NAME	AVERAGE PORTION		
	Measure	Wt./Gms	Calories

FLOWER, FRUIT and SEED VEGETABLES

Name	Measure	Wt./Gms	Calories
Peas, dry, split	1 cup	200	689
Peppers, green, raw	1 medium	76	16
Pumpkin, cnd.	1 cup	228	76
Soybeans, dry	1 cup	210	695
Soybean flour, med. fat	1 cup	88	232
Soybean, sprouts, raw	1 cup	107	50
Squash, summer, frz.	1 cup ckd.	210	44
Squash, winter, ckd.	1 cup mashed	205	97
Succotash, frz.	3/4 cup	210	205
Tomatoes, raw	1 med. 2x2 1/2"	150	30
Tomatoes, cnd.	1 cup	242	46
Tomato ketchup	1 tbsp.	17	17
Tomato puree, cnd.	1 cup	249	90

MISCELLANEOUS

Name	Measure	Wt./Gms	Calories
Beer (4% alcohol)	12 oz.	360	72-173
Coffee, black	1 cup	230	9
Cola beverages	6 oz.	180	83
Ginger ale	6 oz.	180	63
Popcorn	1 cup	14	54
Potato chips	10 medium, 2"	20	180
Yeast, bakers compressed	1 oz.	28	24
Yeast, brewers, dry	1 tbsp.	8	22